The Practical Anti-Inflammatory Diet Guide for Beginners

Easy and Tasty Solutions to Calm Inflammation, Increase Vitality, and Improve Digestion without Breaking the Bank

Caroline Green Chow

Copyright © 2024 by Caroline Green Chow

The content within this book may not be reproduced, duplicated, or transmitted without direct written permission from the author or the publisher.

Under no circumstances will any blame or legal responsibility be held against the publisher, or author, for any damages, reparation, or monetary loss due to the information contained within this book, either directly or indirectly.

Legal Notice:

This book is copyright protected. It is only for personal use. You cannot amend, distribute, sell, use, quote, or paraphrase any part of the content within this book, without the consent of the author or publisher.

Disclaimer Notice:

Please note the information contained within this document is for educational and entertainment purposes only. All effort has been expended to present accurate, up-to-date, reliable, and complete information. No warranties of any kind are declared or implied. Readers acknowledge that the author is not engaged in the rendering of legal, financial, medical, or professional advice. The content within this book has been derived from various sources. Please consult a licensed professional before attempting any techniques outlined in this book.

By reading this document, the reader agrees that under no circumstances is the author responsible for any losses, direct or indirect, that are incurred as a result of the use of the information contained within this document, including, but not limited to, errors, omissions, or inaccuracies.

Contents

Introduction ... 7

1. UNDERSTANDING INFLAMMATION AND ITS IMPACTS ... 11
   What Is Inflammation and Why Should You Care? ... 12
   Chronic versus Acute Inflammation: Recognizing the Differences ... 14
   Common Health Issues Associated with Chronic Inflammation ... 16
   Debunking Myths: The Real Facts about Inflammation ... 18
   How Your Diet Influences Inflammation in Your Body ... 20
   The Science of Anti-Inflammatory Eating: What the Research Says ... 22

2. ANTI-INFLAMMATORY DIET BASICS ... 25
   Key Components of an Anti-Inflammatory Diet ... 25
   Foods to Embrace for Reducing Inflammation ... 28
   Foods to Avoid: What Not to Eat ... 30
   Understanding Food Labels and Inflammatory Additives ... 33
   The Role of Gut Health in Inflammation ... 36
   Balancing Macronutrients for Optimal Health ... 38

3. PRACTICAL MEAL PLANNING AND PREPARATION ... 43
   Designing Your Anti-Inflammatory Meal Plan ... 43
   Grocery Shopping Made Simple: A Buyer's Guide ... 46
   Prepping Meals in Advance: Time-Saving Tips ... 49
   Quick and Easy Anti-Inflammatory Breakfast Ideas ... 52
   Lunches to Reduce Flare-Ups While at Work ... 56
   Simple and Satisfying Anti-Inflammatory Dinners ... 59

4. DELICIOUS RECIPES THAT WON'T BREAK
   THE BANK   63
   Budget-Friendly Anti-Inflammatory Ingredients   63
   Family-Friendly Recipes Everyone Will Love   66
   Comfort Foods: Healthy Twists on Classic Favorites   69
   Snacks and Small Bites for Busy Days   71
   Decadent Desserts without the Guilt   74
   Celebratory Meals and Special Occasions   77

5. OVERCOMING CHALLENGES AND HANDLING
   SETBACKS   81
   Staying on Track during the Holidays   81
   Navigating Social Gatherings and Eating Out   84
   Dealing with Cravings and Temptations   86
   How to Modify Your Favorite Recipes   88
   Addressing Common Dietary Concerns and Missteps   91
   Reassessing and Adjusting Your Diet over Time   93

6. BEYOND DIET: LIFESTYLE CHANGES FOR
   MANAGING INFLAMMATION   99
   The Importance of Regular Physical Activity   99
   Stress Reduction Techniques That Work   101
   The Impact of Sleep on Inflammation   104
   Hydration: Your Secret Weapon Against
   Inflammation   106
   Supplements and Natural Remedies   108
   Building a Support System for Long-Term Success   110

7. ADVANCED TOPICS IN ANTI-INFLAMMATORY
   LIVING   113
   The Truth about Nightshades and Inflammation   113
   Alcohol and Inflammation: What You Need to Know   115
   Dairy: Friend or Foe in an Anti-Inflammatory Diet?   117
   The Role of Fats: Omega-3s versus Omega-6s   120
   Understanding Food Intolerances and Allergies   122
   The Power of Spices and Herbs in Your Diet   124

8. MOTIVATION AND REAL-LIFE SUCCESS
   STORIES   129
   Inspiring Stories from Those Who've Made the
   Change   130
   Tips for Staying Motivated on Your Health Journey   132

The Role of Community in Lifestyle Change	135
Celebrating Your Successes: Milestones and Rewards	137
Adjusting Your Mindset for Health and Wellness	139
Encouraging Family and Friends to Join You on Your Journey	141
Conclusion	145
9. BONUS CHAPTER WITH ADDITIONAL RECIPES	149
List of Recipes for Comfort Foods	149
List of Recipes for One-Pot Dishes	150
Recipes: Anti-Inflammatory Comfort Foods	150
Recipes: One-Pot Dishes	185
References and Resources	201

Introduction

Every year, millions grapple with the persistent ache and discomfort of chronic inflammation, often feeling trapped in a cycle of medication and temporary remedies. But there's hope. Take, for instance, Sarah, a middle-aged schoolteacher whose daily battle with joint pain and fatigue seemed endless. Traditional treatments brought little relief, and her quality of life was slipping away until she discovered the transformative potential of the anti-inflammatory diet—a journey that not only alleviated her symptoms but also revitalized her entire approach to eating and wellness, offering a beacon of hope and relief for those in similar situations.

What exactly is an anti-inflammatory diet? At its core, it's a method of choosing and cooking foods based on scientific knowledge of how such foods can help your body maintain optimum health. For instance, you should concentrate on incorporating whole, nutrient-dense foods like leafy greens, fatty fish, and berries that combat inflammation into your diet while avoiding foods like processed meats, refined sugars, and trans fats, which are known inflammation triggers.

This guide emerged from my struggle with chronic inflammation. Faced with the limitations of traditional remedies, I found solace and significant improvement through dietary changes. The impact was so profound that I felt compelled to share what I had learned. This guide isn't just a collection of recipes; it's a lifeline to anyone seeking a sustainable path to better health through mindful eating.

On these pages, you will find more than meal plans and recipes. This guide is designed to offer practical, affordable, and scientifically backed advice on taming inflammation. Whether you're a busy parent, a student, or someone simply trying to balance health with a hectic schedule, the solutions here are crafted to fit into your life seamlessly.

What sets this book apart is its commitment to realism and accessibility. It's packed with strategies for incorporating the anti-inflammatory diet into daily life, including holidays and special occasions, and emphasizes using ingredients that don't break the bank. Plus, it provides information about the helpful high-tech tools to make your journey interactive, from apps that help track your progress to websites offering supportive communities. This practical and affordable approach is designed to reassure you that managing inflammation is not only possible but also within reach.

I'll also address the top ten myths about inflammation, providing you with the facts you need to make informed health decisions. This book is more than just informative—it's motivational. It includes stories of people who have significantly improved their health and well-being through the anti-inflammatory diet. These anecdotes serve as proof of the diet's efficacy and as encouragement that this lifestyle change is achievable and rewarding.

I invite you to use this book as a tool for your health journey. Engage with the interactive elements, such as meal planning templates, shopping lists, and progress trackers, and tailor the action plans to fit your needs. This book is your path to empowerment, a guide designed to equip you with the knowledge and confidence to manage your inflammation and elevate your overall health. With this guide, you can take control of your health and be confident in your ability to make a positive change.

Let's take these steps together toward a healthier, more vibrant life.

Understanding Inflammation and Its Impacts

Have you ever woken up feeling like your body can't get moving or perhaps noticed that some days, your joints and muscles inexplicably ache more than usual? It's easy to dismiss these signals as just part of a bad day or the unavoidable toll of aging. However, these could very well be signs of inflammation in your body—a condition that, if left unchecked, can shift from being a fleeting visitor to an unwelcome long-term resident, impacting your health in myriad ways.

Inflammation is often discussed in a negative light, but it's not all bad. It's your body's frontline defense system, a crucial part of the healing process. However, when inflammation lingers longer than necessary, it can lead to many problems. This chapter will guide you through understanding the dual faces of inflammation—how it can be both a protector and a potential threat. By the end of this section, you'll have a clearer picture of why a proactive approach to managing inflammation can be a game-changer for your health and well-being.

What Is Inflammation and Why Should You Care?

Definition and Biological Role

Inflammation is your body's knee-jerk response to injury or infection. Think of it as your biological security system that springs into action whenever there's a threat to your body's equilibrium. When triggered, a flurry of immune activity occurs, aiming to remove harmful stimuli, including damaged cells, irritants, or pathogens. Subsequently, the body initiates the healing process.

This protective mechanism is essential; wounds wouldn't heal without it, and infections could become deadly. The typical signs of acute inflammation—redness, heat, swelling, pain, and sometimes loss of function—are the visible manifestations of your immune system at work. Increased blood flow to the affected area causes redness and heat. Swelling occurs as fluids accumulate to help ferry immune cells to where they're needed most, and pain is a signal that something's wrong, often prompting us to reduce further harm to the area by limiting movement or use.

Symptoms and Signs

You've likely experienced the symptoms of inflammation firsthand during illnesses like the flu or physical injuries like sprained ankles. These are classic signs of acute inflammation, where the body focuses its healing efforts on a particular area. It's your body telling you it's fighting off invaders and repairing itself. While uncomfortable, these signs are temporary and resolve as your body heals.

Long-Term Effects

Yet, if inflammation lingers and shifts into a chronic state, it ceases to be beneficial. Instead, it acts like a persistent ember, slowly inflicting damage on your body. This prolonged state of inflammation subtly paves the way for a host of diseases, including arthritis, heart disease, and certain types of cancer. Over time, chronic inflammation can wreak havoc on your DNA and disrupt cellular functions, impairing essential bodily processes that are necessary for maintaining health.

Relevance to Daily Life

Understanding inflammation and effectively managing it involves more than just taking medication to reduce symptoms. Your lifestyle choices, particularly your diet, play pivotal roles in influencing inflammation levels. Your daily habits, which include exercise and the stress levels you face, play a crucial role in either dampening or intensifying inflammation. Therefore, it's essential to adopt habits that support a balanced inflammatory response. By choosing anti-inflammatory foods and maintaining an active, stress-managed lifestyle, you can significantly reduce the risk of chronic inflammation and its unwelcome consequences.

In this chapter, we will explore how simple, deliberate choices in your daily life can help manage and mitigate chronic inflammation. You'll learn to make informed decisions that enhance your body's natural defenses, improve your overall health, and empower you to lead a vibrant, active life free from the pain and limitations of unchecked inflammation.

Chronic versus Acute Inflammation: Recognizing the Differences

To truly grasp the impact of inflammation on your health, it's essential to distinguish between its two primary forms—acute and chronic. Acute inflammation is the body's immediate response to an injury or infection. It's intense and short-lived, serving a crucial role in healing and protection. Consider the reaction when you accidentally touch a hot stove; the swift onset of redness and swelling is your body deploying fluids and white blood cells to the affected area, initiating the healing process. This type of inflammation is vital; it's your body's way of saying, "Hey, something's wrong here," and without it, wounds would fester, and infections could spiral out of control.

Conversely, chronic inflammation is a more subtle yet harmful condition that can go unnoticed for an extended period. It diverges from the acute variety because it doesn't serve the body's repair mechanisms. Instead, it's akin to a lingering fire that, instead of aiding in recovery, begins to damage the body from within. While this type of inflammation may present less dramatically, its prolonged presence poses a greater risk to our health. Consider a scenario in which you're constantly exposed to low levels of pollution or stress. While these may not induce the pronounced response characteristic of acute inflammation, they can maintain your body's inflammatory mechanisms in a constant, albeit mild, state of activation. Over time, this contributes to chronic inflammation, placing the body in an ongoing, low-grade state of alert, mistakenly perceiving a threat where none exists.

The distinction between these two types of inflammation is critical because each impacts health differently. While occasionally severe, acute inflammation is self-limiting, meaning it resolves when the injury heals or the infection clears. Chronic inflammation, however, does not shut off. It lingers and can silently damage tissues and organs, sometimes for years, without the overt symptoms that characterize acute inflammation. For instance, while the acute inflammation of a sprained ankle will cause redness and swelling that goes away with time, the chronic inflammation associated with an autoimmune disease like rheumatoid arthritis persists, causing joint damage and pain that can last a lifetime.

Recognizing whether inflammation is acute or chronic is vital because it can influence your decisions about how to manage your health. If you understand that the swelling and redness from stubbing your toe is just your body healing itself, you're less likely to panic and more likely to give it the care it needs. Conversely, knowing that the persistent, low-grade discomfort you feel isn't just a series of bad days but chronic inflammation may prompt you to make lifestyle changes that could significantly impact your long-term health. Such changes include adjusting your diet to include more anti-inflammatory foods, incorporating regular exercise into your routine, and managing stress effectively—all of which can help turn the tide against chronic inflammation and improve your overall well-being.

This understanding empowers you to take proactive steps toward managing your health, emphasizing the importance of lifestyle choices in maintaining an optimal balance within your body. By keeping inflammation in check, you're not just avoiding pain or discomfort but actively contributing to a healthier, more vibrant life. This proactive approach is not about quick fixes or temporary remedies; it's about making sustainable changes that enhance your body's resilience against the stresses that can trigger inflammation.

Common Health Issues Associated with Chronic Inflammation

When we discuss chronic inflammation, it's essential to understand that its impact stretches far beyond temporary discomfort or swelling—it's a pervasive condition that can influence the entire body, often in ways that aren't immediately apparent. Chronic inflammation acts as a silent alarm that, if ignored, can contribute to the development of several major health conditions. These conditions include heart disease, diabetes, cancer, and Alzheimer's disease, each associated with heightened inflammatory responses over prolonged periods.

Heart disease, for instance, is intricately linked to inflammation in the cardiovascular system. When blood vessels remain inflamed, it can lead to atherosclerosis, in which plaque builds up, narrowing arteries and increasing the risk of heart attacks and strokes. Similarly, in type 2 diabetes, chronic inflammation affects the body's ability to manage insulin, eventually leading to insulin resistance and impaired glucose tolerance. With cancer, the scenario is a bit more complex. Here, inflammation contributes to various cellular processes that support the proliferation, growth, and survival of malignant cells. Moreover, Alzheimer's disease is now often referred to as "type 3 diabetes" due to its links with inflammatory processes that damage neurons and disrupt brain function.

The signs of chronic inflammation can be diverse and, regrettably, are often subtle enough to be mistaken for symptoms of other conditions, leading them to be frequently ignored. Persistent fatigue that doesn't seem to go away with rest, digestive issues like constipation, diarrhea, and abdominal pain, or more frequent infections can all signal that your body is dealing with low-grade, persistent inflammation. Recognizing these signs early is important in preventing the progression of inflammation-related conditions.

Consider the case of John, a fifty-eight-year-old office worker with a family history of heart disease. For years, John battled with subtle symptoms like mild joint pain and occasional digestive upset—symptoms that are easy to dismiss in a busy life. It wasn't until a routine check-up revealed elevated markers of inflammation that John realized these were not just random occurrences. This wake-up call led him to modify his lifestyle drastically, incorporating anti-inflammatory foods and regular exercise into his daily routine. Over time, not only did his symptoms improve, but his biomarkers for inflammation significantly decreased, exemplifying how understanding and addressing chronic inflammation can pivotally influence health outcomes.

Preventing these diseases and managing chronic inflammation doesn't require drastic changes overnight but involves consistent, manageable adjustments to lifestyle and diet. Incorporating anti-inflammatory foods like leafy greens, nuts, fatty fish, and whole grains can make a significant difference. Equally, reducing the intake of processed foods, sugars, and unhealthy fats is essential. Physical activity plays a dual role—it directly reduces inflammatory markers and helps in weight management, which can further reduce the burden of inflammation. Managing stress is also a critical component in controlling inflammation. Adopting practices like yoga, meditation, or simple breathing techniques plays an essential role in mitigating the body's stress hormones. These hormones often initiate inflammatory responses, so managing stress through these activities can further dampen the flames of inflammation.

Understanding the deep connection between chronic inflammation and prevalent health issues underscores the importance of proactive health management. By tuning into your body's signals and making informed choices about diet, exercise, and stress reduction, you empower yourself to lead a healthier life, minimizing the risk of inflammation-driven diseases. This proactive stance is not just about preventing disease but enhancing the overall quality of life, ensuring that your later years are more numerous, more vibrant, and more fulfilling.

Debunking Myths: The Real Facts about Inflammation

In a world brimming with information and just as many misconceptions, it's crucial to separate fact from fiction, particularly when it comes to your health. Inflammation, often misunderstood, has gathered a host of myths around it—some of which may lead you astray from effective management strategies. Let's clear the air and set the record straight on some of the most common myths about inflammation, providing you with the knowledge to make informed decisions about your health and lifestyle.

One prevalent myth is the blanket statement that "all inflammation is bad." As we've explored, inflammation is fundamentally a protective response, crucial for healing wounds and fending off infections. Chronic, unchecked inflammation poses a problem, not acute, temporary inflammation, which occurs when you cut your finger or sprain an ankle. Understanding this distinction is vital because it influences how you respond to inflammation. For example, anti-inflammatory medications to suppress acute inflammation can delay healing. Therefore, it's not about eliminating inflammation indiscriminately but managing it wisely to support the body's natural healing process.

Diet also plays a significant role in managing inflammation, yet here too, myths abound. A common misconception is that certain "superfoods" can miraculously cure inflammation. While it's true that foods like turmeric, ginger, and omega-3-rich foods have anti-inflammatory properties, no single food is a magic bullet. Inflammation management is most effective when approached holistically. Including a variety of these foods in a balanced diet is more beneficial than relying on one superfood. Embracing this approach ensures that your actions transcend simply addressing inflammation; it cultivates overall health by supplying a wide variety of necessary nutrients.

When it comes to supplements, another area rife with misconceptions, it's essential to tread carefully. Many believe taking high doses of anti-inflammatory supplements like fish oil or curcumin can substitute for dietary and lifestyle changes. However, supplements should complement, not replace, a healthy diet and lifestyle. While they can help manage inflammation, they are most effective when used in conjunction with other healthy habits. For instance, a high-quality fish oil supplement may help reduce inflammation. However, its benefits are greatly enhanced when you also reduce the intake of pro-inflammatory foods, like processed meats and refined sugars.

Finally, let's address the myth that minimal exercise does not impact inflammation levels. Current research suggests quite the opposite. Regular, moderate exercise has been shown to lower inflammation over time. It can help reduce the levels of inflammatory markers, such as C-reactive protein (CRP), and boost the production of anti-inflammatory compounds within the body. Even activities as simple as brisk walking or cycling can have profound anti-inflammatory effects when performed regularly. This fact underscores the importance of incorporating physical activity into your routine, no matter how minimal it might seem. Every bit counts in the fight against chronic inflammation.

Understanding these truths helps demystify inflammation and guides more effective management through diet, lifestyle adjustments, and proper use of supplements. Armed with accurate insights, you can confidently navigate choices that tackle inflammation head-on and enhance your overall well-being. It's important to remember that the aim isn't to fight inflammation at every turn but instead to harmonize your body's reactions, nurturing an environment that promotes vitality and robust health. Adopting a holistic strategy allows you to transform inflammation from a persistent foe into a beneficial partner in your journey toward healing.

How Your Diet Influences Inflammation in Your Body

Understanding how your diet impacts inflammation in your body is paramount for anyone looking to improve their health through nutritional choices. The foods you eat may either contribute to an inflammatory state or help alleviate it. In this section, we'll explore how certain foods can provoke inflammatory responses while others can be incredibly beneficial in reducing inflammation. Additionally, I'll share practical tips on how to weave anti-inflammatory foods into your everyday meals, ensuring your meals taste good and support your overall health.

Let's start with pro-inflammatory foods, which can significantly contribute to chronic inflammation when excessive amounts are consumed. Processed sugars and trans fats are prime culprits here. Foods high in processed sugars, such as soft drinks, candies, and even some cereals, can rapidly increase blood sugar levels. This spike causes the body to release pro-inflammatory messengers called cytokines. Trans fats, found in many fried foods, baked goods, and processed snacks, are known to raise LDL (aka bad) cholesterol levels and lower HDL (aka good) cholesterol levels, promoting inflammation. These fats can also trigger endothelial dysfunction, a condition where the blood vessels become less efficient at regulating blood flow, further contributing to inflammatory processes.

On the flip side, integrating anti-inflammatory foods into your daily eating plan can serve as a powerful strategy to mitigate inflammation. Foods rich in omega-3 fatty acids, such as salmon, flaxseeds, and walnuts, are known for their ability to reduce inflammation. Omega-3 fatty acids compete with pro-inflammatory omega-6 fatty acids (found in many vegetable oils) for use in the body's biochemical pathways. By balancing the ratio of omega-3 to omega-6, you can reduce the production of inflammatory substances. Additionally, incorporating foods rich in antioxidants is a key strategy for fighting inflammation. Antioxidants counteract the effects of free radicals, which are unstable molecules that can lead to oxidative stress and inflammation in the body. Antioxidant-rich foods such as berries, leafy greens, nuts, and seeds reduce inflammation and protect your health by neutralizing these harmful molecules. Foods abundant in antioxidants play a crucial role in combating inflammation by neutralizing free radicals. This approach effectively reduces bodily inflammation.

The importance of a balanced diet in managing inflammation cannot be overstated. Rather than focusing on single nutrients, a holistic approach to diet is most beneficial. This approach means diversifying your diet with a wide array of foods to ensure a comprehensive nutrient profile that supports an anti-inflammatory state in the body. A diet emphasizing whole, nutrient-dense foods over processed options forms the cornerstone of anti-inflammatory eating. It does not mean you must overhaul your diet overnight or swear off treats. It is about making more mindful daily choices, gradually shifting toward foods that nourish and protect your body.

For those looking to integrate anti-inflammatory foods into their diet, start simple. Incorporate more fruits and vegetables into each meal; they're rich in antioxidants and fiber, which has been shown to reduce inflammatory responses. Switch out refined grains for whole grains like quinoa, barley, and oats, which contain higher fiber and nutrient content, playing a pivotal role in managing inflammation. Instead of cooking with butter or vegetable oils high in omega-6 fatty acids, opt for olive oil or avocado oil. These oils are better for heart health and can help reduce inflammation. Small, consistent changes like these can significantly affect how you feel.

Making these dietary changes doesn't require extraordinary effort or expense. Start by adding one anti-inflammatory food to each meal and gradually build from there. Snack on nuts instead of chips, add berries to your breakfast cereal, or choose fish twice a week instead of red meat. Remember, the goal is to make sustainable changes that enhance your health without feeling restrictive. Emphasizing a diet enriched with an assortment of whole foods and limiting processed food consumption can markedly diminish inflammation, thereby improving your overall health and vitality.

The Science of Anti-Inflammatory Eating: What the Research Says

The correlation between diet and inflammation has been a focal point of numerous scientific studies over the past decades. These investigations have shed light on how certain dietary patterns can significantly affect markers of inflammation in the body. For instance, time and again, studies have highlighted that consuming a diet rich in fruits, vegetables, nuts, whole grains, fish, and beneficial oils can significantly diminish inflammation levels. These foods can improve markers such as C-reactive protein (CRP), interleukin-6 (IL-6), and tumor necrosis factor-alpha (TNFα). These findings reinforce the importance of diet in managing inflammation and guide us in making informed choices about the foods we eat.

Specific nutrients have been identified for their roles in reducing inflammation. Polyphenols, for example, are compounds found abundantly in natural plant food sources such as berries, tea, dark chocolate, wine, and certain fruits and vegetables. The anti-inflammatory effects of polyphenols are due to their ability to modify inflammation-producing processes in the body. They interfere with the production of inflammatory cytokines and enhance the production of anti-inflammatory cytokines. Flavonoids, a specific type of polyphenol, are found in fruits, vegetables, grains, bark, roots, stems, flowers, tea, and wine. They play a similar role by inhibiting enzymes involved in synthesizing inflammatory substances, thus acting as powerful anti-inflammatory agents.

The impact of whole dietary patterns on inflammation has been particularly illuminating. The Mediterranean diet, which is high in fruits, vegetables, nuts, whole grains, fish, and olive oil, is associated with lower levels of inflammatory markers. This diet highlights foods rich in omega-3 fatty acids, antioxidants, and polyphenols, which are known for their anti-inflammatory effects. Similarly, plant-based diets, which are high in fiber, antioxidants, and other phytochemicals, have been shown to reduce inflammation. Research comparing plant-based diets with Western diets rich in processed and animal products has consistently demonstrated a lower prevalence of inflammatory markers in those following plant-based dietary patterns.

However, it's important to acknowledge gaps in the existing research. While the link between diet and inflammation is well established, many studies are observational, which can show associations but not prove causation. Consequently, there is a need for more controlled trials to understand fully the mechanisms by which diet influences inflammation. Additionally, most research has been conducted in Western populations, with less focus on how these findings might translate to other cultural groups who may have different dietary patterns and genetic predispositions to inflammation-related diseases.

This evolving field of research underscores the potential of diet as a powerful tool in preventing and managing inflammation. By understanding the roles specific nutrients and dietary patterns play in influencing inflammation, individuals can make more informed choices about their diets. These choices have the potential to reduce their risk of chronic diseases related to high levels of inflammation. As research unfolds, it will provide a clearer, more detailed map of the intricate interactions between our diet and inflammation, guiding us toward more effective strategies for maintaining our health and well-being.

Anti-Inflammatory Diet Basics

Imagine walking into a vibrant market where every stall offers a feast for the eyes and the promise of health—fruits bursting with juice, nuts, seeds rich in oils, and whole grains that tell a story of the earth's generosity. This is what adopting an anti-inflammatory diet can feel like—an exploration of natural foods that are not only delicious but inherently packed with properties that can calm and prevent inflammation. This chapter is your guide to understanding these foods and how to integrate them into your daily life, ensuring every meal is a step toward better health.

Key Components of an Anti-Inflammatory Diet

Whole Foods Focus

The cornerstone of an anti-inflammatory diet is the emphasis on whole, unprocessed foods. Whole foods are those that have been minimally altered from their natural state. They do not contain the added sugars, fats, and preservatives that are common in processed foods, which are known to trigger inflammatory responses in the body. More importantly, whole foods retain their natural composition, including a host of anti-inflammatory compounds such as antioxidants, phytonutrients, vitamins, and minerals. These components are often lost or diminished during processing. When shopping, look for foods that are as close to their natural state as possible, such as fresh fruits and vegetables, lean proteins, and whole grains.

For example, consider a whole apple versus commercially produced apple juice. The whole apple contains fiber, vitamins, and other compounds that work together to reduce inflammation. The juice, however, often lacks fiber and includes added sugars, which can increase inflammation. Similarly, processed foods like sugary cereals, white bread, and fast food often contain high levels of added sugars, unhealthy fats, and preservatives, all of which can trigger inflammation. By choosing whole foods and avoiding these processed options, you're not just nourishing your body; you're actively fighting against the processes that lead to chronic inflammation.

Variety

Incorporating a diverse range of foods is crucial in an anti-inflammatory diet. Each type of food brings its unique anti-inflammatory properties to the table. For instance, leafy greens are rich in vitamin K and several antioxidants, fatty fish are high in omega-3 fatty acids, and berries offer a wide range of phenolic compounds, all known for their anti-inflammatory effects. Eating a variety of these foods ensures you get a comprehensive array of nutrients that work together to combat inflammation. This diversity not only applies to the types of foods but also to colors. The concept of "eating the rainbow" refers to the idea that foods of different colors often provide different nutrients—such as the lycopene in red tomatoes or the anthocyanins in blueberries. By adding a variety of colorful foods to your plate, you're not only making your meals visually appealing but also ensuring a broad intake of essential nutrients that support overall health.

Moderation and Balance

While it's essential to incorporate healthy, anti-inflammatory foods into your diet, balance and moderation are key. Even too much of a good thing can be harmful. For instance, while nuts are excellent sources of healthy fats and proteins, they are also high in calories. Consuming them in excessive amounts could lead to weight gain, which is considered a risk factor for inflammation. Balancing your food intake involves understanding portion sizes and listening to your body's hunger and fullness cues. Achieving this balance entails not confining your diet too strictly to certain foods but exploring ways to incorporate a broad spectrum of nutrients. This balance ensures that you do not consume too many calories while still getting the adequate nutrition your body needs to combat inflammation.

Regular Meal Times

Eating at regular intervals can play a significant role in managing inflammation. Consistent meal timing helps regulate your body's metabolic processes, including insulin production and fat metabolism, which can help manage inflammation. Irregular eating patterns can disrupt these processes and can lead to increased inflammation. Furthermore, regular meal times can also help improve your digestion and overall metabolism. Maintaining a meal schedule enhances your body's ability to process and assimilate nutrients, bolstering your defenses against inflammation.

Incorporating these elements into your daily eating habits can transform your approach to meals from mere consumption to intentionally nurturing your body. As you continue to explore the depths of the anti-inflammatory diet, remember that each food choice is an opportunity to influence your health positively. Your diet does not just impact your momentary cravings but plays a crucial role in shaping your long-term wellness trajectory. By focusing on whole foods, embracing variety, practicing moderation, and maintaining regular meal times, you are laying the foundations of a diet that combats inflammation and supports a vibrant, energetic life.

Foods to Embrace for Reducing Inflammation

Certain foods act as powerful allies in your quest to quell inflammation and enhance your overall health. Among these, fatty fish such as salmon and mackerel are standout choices due to their high levels of omega-3 fatty acids. Additionally, plant-based sources such as flaxseeds, chia seeds and walnuts are rich in omega-3 fatty acids. These essential fats are well-known for their anti-inflammatory properties. Omega-3s help reduce the production of inflammatory eicosanoids and cytokines, which are biochemicals that can contribute to inflammation in the body. Regular consumption of these fish or plant-based sources can lead to significant decreases in the levels of inflammatory markers such as C-reactive protein (CRP) and interleukin-6 (IL-6). A simple way to incorporate these into your diet is by planning a couple of meals each week that feature fatty fish or seeds and nuts with omega-3 fatty acids. Not only is this practice beneficial for your inflammatory response, but it also supports heart health and cognitive function.

In the plant kingdom, colorful fruits and vegetables present a spectrum of anti-inflammatory benefits, primarily due to their high antioxidant content. Foods such as berries, oranges, and leafy greens are rich in vitamins and phytochemicals that fight oxidative stress, a key contributor to inflammation. For instance, berries contain anthocyanins, potent antioxidants that have been observed to reduce inflammation markers in the body. Similarly, the vibrant orange color of carrots and sweet potatoes is from beta-carotene, another powerful antioxidant. Including a variety of colorful fruits and vegetables in your diet helps reduce inflammation and ensures a broad intake of essential nutrients that support overall health.

Nuts and seeds are another group of foods beneficial for their anti-inflammatory properties. Almonds, flaxseeds, and chia seeds are excellent sources of alpha-linolenic acid (ALA), a type of plant-based omega-3 fatty acid. ALA helps mitigate inflammation and has been linked to a lower risk of chronic diseases such as heart disease and arthritis. These seeds and nuts are also high in fiber. Foods that are high in fiber can help reduce inflammation by promoting a healthy gut microbiome. A simple way to include more nuts and seeds in your diet is by adding them to your oatmeal or yogurt in the mornings, blending them into smoothies, or using them as a crunchy salad topping. Their addition enhances the texture and flavor of your meals and boosts their nutritional profile.

Lastly, the culinary world offers many herbs and spices known for their anti-inflammatory effects. Turmeric, for example, contains curcumin, a compound with potent anti-inflammatory and antioxidant properties. Studies have indicated that curcumin can influence several biological processes involved in inflammation, pain, and swelling. To incorporate turmeric into your diet, you can simply add the spice to smoothies, soups, or curries. Ginger and garlic also offer substantial anti-inflammatory benefits. Ginger reduces inflammation by inhibiting the synthesis of pro-inflammatory prostaglandins, while garlic's sulfur compounds can suppress the pathways that lead to inflammatory processes. Adding these spices to your daily meals does more than improve the flavor—it also strengthens your dietary defense against inflammation.

Each food group offers unique and powerful benefits that can help manage and reduce inflammation. By adding fatty fish, a variety of colorful fruits and vegetables, nuts and seeds, and a range of herbs and spices to your diet, you enrich the flavors of your meals and take a decisive step toward mitigating chronic inflammation and embracing a healthier lifestyle. This approach to eating emphasizes natural, nutrient-rich foods that support your body's health on multiple levels, aligning with your goals of leading a vibrant, active life free from the discomfort of inflammation.

Foods to Avoid: What Not to Eat

Navigating the world of anti-inflammatory eating isn't just about piling your plate with beneficial foods; equally important is avoiding foods that can intensify inflammation. Understanding what not to eat is crucial because inflammatory foods can counteract the benefits of your healthy selections. In this part of our guide, we spotlight some of the major culprits that can provoke inflammatory responses in your body—processed foods, refined sugars, certain fats and oils, and excessive alcohol. By learning why these substances can be harmful and how to avoid them, you'll be better equipped to maintain an anti-inflammatory diet that truly benefits your health.

Processed Foods

Highly processed foods often contain ingredients that promote inflammation, such as excess salt, sugar, and unhealthy fats. These foods, which include most packaged snacks, fast foods, and ready-to-eat meals, undergo extensive processing, which strips away beneficial nutrients like fiber and replaces them with preservatives and flavor enhancers. The problem with these additives and altered ingredients is that they can trigger a series of inflammatory reactions in the body. For instance, excessive salts can lead to water retention and high blood pressure, straining your circulatory system and fostering inflammation. Meanwhile, the artificial additives often found in these foods can disrupt your gut microbiome, an essential element of your immune system, thus facilitating an inflammatory environment. Opting for fresh, minimally processed foods not only diminishes your intake of these inflammatory compounds but also enhances your consumption of natural anti-inflammatory agents found in whole foods.

Refined Sugars

The impact of refined sugars on your body's inflammatory processes is particularly stark. Foods high in refined sugars, such as sodas, pastries, and many dessert items, can quickly spike blood sugar levels. This spike prompts your body to release insulin in large amounts, a response that can trigger the production of inflammatory cytokines. Moreover, high blood sugar levels can cause advanced glycation end products (AGEs)—harmful compounds that can further stimulate inflammation—to be produced. To mitigate these effects, consider natural sweeteners like honey or maple syrup. They have a lower glycemic index and contain antioxidants that can help fight inflammation. Additionally, integrating fruits into your diet as a source of natural sweetness is an excellent way to satisfy sugar cravings without the inflammatory response associated with refined sugars.

Trans Fats and Certain Oils

Trans fats are among the most inflammatory foods you can consume. Trans fats are found in fried foods, baked goods, and processed snacks. They can increase LDL (aka bad) cholesterol levels while decreasing HDL (aka good) cholesterol, fostering inflammation throughout the cardiovascular system. Moreover, these fats can promote insulin resistance, further contributing to inflammatory processes. It's also essential to be cautious with vegetable oils high in omega-6 fatty acids, like corn and safflower. While omega-6 fats are necessary in small amounts, excessive consumption can lead to an imbalance between omega-6 and omega-3 fatty acids, exacerbating inflammatory responses. Choosing oils that are high in omega-3 fatty acids—such as flaxseed oil—or making a switch to olive oil, renowned for its high content of anti-inflammatory monounsaturated fats, is an effective strategy to restore the balance between omega-6 and omega-3 fatty acids and diminish inflammation.

Excessive Alcohol

Moderation is crucial when it comes to alcohol consumption. Excessive alcohol intake has been linked to increased inflammation. High levels of alcohol can disrupt the balance of the gut microbiome, impairing your body's ability to regulate inflammation and protect against bacteria. Alcohol metabolism also produces acetaldehyde, a toxic compound that can damage liver cells, promoting inflammation.

You can significantly influence your body's inflammatory status by making informed choices about what to avoid and what to embrace in your diet. Steering clear of processed foods, refined sugars, unhealthy fats, and alcohol can help maintain the benefits of the nutrient-rich, anti-inflammatory foods you incorporate into your daily meals. This proactive approach to diet management supports overall health and enhances quality of life by reducing the risk of inflammation-related health issues.

Understanding Food Labels and Inflammatory Additives

Walking through the aisles of modern grocery stores without the proper knowledge can feel like navigating a minefield, especially for those aiming to diminish inflammation through their diet. The shelves brim with attractive products, but some products are laced with hidden ingredients that could harm your health. Learning to read and interpret food labels is like having a guide in this complex terrain, enabling you to make choices that align with your health objectives.

When examining food labels, the first step is to look beyond the marketing claims on the front of the package. In the U.S., phrases like "all-natural" or "healthy" are not regulated strictly and can be misleading. Instead, focus on the ingredient list and nutrition facts panel. Ingredients are typically listed in descending order by weight, which means the first few ingredients are what the product is mainly made of. Be wary of long lists containing unfamiliar or unpronounceable items—these are often additives that could promote inflammation.

Among the most common inflammatory additives to avoid are MSG (monosodium glutamate), artificial sweeteners, and various preservatives. MSG is often hidden under other names, such as hydrolyzed vegetable protein or yeast extract, and can trigger inflammatory responses, particularly in sensitive individuals. While calorie-free, artificial sweeteners like aspartame and sucralose can disrupt gut health and insulin sensitivity, indirectly promoting inflammation. Preservatives like sodium benzoate and butylated hydroxyanisole (BHA) are added to extend shelf life but can adversely affect immune function and encourage inflammatory processes. By learning to identify these additives on labels, you can steer clear of products that may aggravate inflammation, opting instead for cleaner, more wholesome options.

Importance of Organic Foods

Often, the debate over choosing organic foods centers around their potential benefits in reducing exposure to pesticides and synthetic chemicals, which are known to contribute to inflammation. Farmers grow organic foods without artificial pesticides and fertilizers, and as a result, the foods tend to have higher nutrient levels and lower pesticide residues. Reducing the chemical load on your body is crucial for managing inflammation, as these substances can contribute to oxidative stress and inflammation. While organic foods may be more expensive, their benefits for health and the environment may justify the cost for those particularly sensitive to chemicals or concerned about long-term health impacts.

For instance, studies have indicated that organic produce can have higher levels of antioxidants than conventionally grown variants.

Antioxidants are crucial in fighting inflammation, as they neutralize free radicals that can cause cellular damage in the body. Additionally, organic farming practices often promote soil health and biodiversity, which can lead to better nutritional profiles for produce. While the decision to go organic is a personal one, replacing some foods with their organic variants—particularly those known to have higher pesticide residues like apples, strawberries, and spinach—can be a beneficial step toward reducing your inflammation load.

Practical Shopping Tips

Effective grocery shopping for an anti-inflammatory diet extends beyond just avoiding certain foods and additives. It's about making strategic choices that maximize nutrient intake without compromising quality or budget. Start by planning for your meals during the coming week and create a shopping list based on these plans. This approach helps ensure you only buy what you need, reducing the temptation to purchase unhealthy foods impulsively.

When shopping, stay on the perimeter of the store as much as possible. This location is typically where the fresh produce, meats, and dairy are, while the aisles in the middle often contain more processed items. When venturing into the aisles, be vigilant and read labels carefully. Look for products with short ingredient lists comprising recognizable foods. Another tip is to shop at local farmers' markets when possible. There, the produce is fresher and typically grown with fewer harsh pesticides. Additionally, shopping there offers the unique benefit of being able to discuss growing practices directly with the farmers.

Including frozen fruits and vegetables in your meal planning is a savvy choice. These items are typically harvested at their nutritional peak and immediately frozen, locking in their vital nutrients and antioxidants. Opting for frozen produce offers a practical and economical way to access nutritious foods year-round. It ensures you're continually fueling your body with anti-inflammatory benefits, regardless of the season. Frozen produce is a cost-effective and convenient way to enjoy fruits and vegetables that may be out of season, ensuring you have a steady supply of anti-inflammatory foods all year round.

By becoming skilled at reading food labels, understanding the implications of additives, and making informed choices about organic produce, you can confidently navigate the grocery store. Mastering these skills transcends simple compliance with an anti-inflammatory diet; it empowers you to take control of your health through each dietary choice you make. As you continue to apply these practices, you'll find that shopping for a diet that supports your well-being becomes easier, more effective, and enjoyable as each choice brings you closer to better health and vitality.

The Role of Gut Health in Inflammation

A healthy gut is often described as the cornerstone of overall wellness, and its role in managing inflammation is crucial. The gut microbiome, which is the vast community of microorganisms living in your digestive system, profoundly impacts your body's immune response and its ability to handle inflammation. These microbes interact with your body's cells to promote healthy immune function and protect against harmful pathogens. When this microbiome is balanced, it supports the body's natural anti-inflammatory responses. However, an imbalance, known as dysbiosis, can lead to increased gut permeability, often called leaky gut, allowing bacterial endotoxins to get into the bloodstream and trigger systemic inflammation.

Supporting gut health, therefore, is an essential strategy for managing inflammation. Probiotics and prebiotics play pivotal roles in this regard. Probiotics are considered beneficial bacteria that help balance the gut microbiome, enhancing its function and reducing inflammatory responses. Probiotics can be found in fermented foods, including yogurt and kefir, which introduce helpful bacteria directly into your digestive system. These foods help populate your gut with beneficial microbes that can outcompete harmful bacteria and reduce inflammation. Supplements are also an option if dietary sources are insufficient or if specific strains of bacteria are needed.

Prebiotics, on the other hand, serve as food for these beneficial bacteria. They are found in fiber-rich foods such as bananas, onions, garlic, and the skins of apples. These nutrients help nourish the good bacteria in your gut, enabling them to thrive and exert their beneficial effects on gut health and inflammation. By combining probiotics with prebiotics, you can create a gut environment that is conducive to maintaining a balanced immune response and managing inflammation effectively.

The role of dietary fiber extends beyond just serving as nourishment for gut bacteria. Fiber has been shown to play a direct role in reducing gut inflammation. This reduction occurs as the gut microbiota ferments the fiber, leading to the production of short-chain fatty acids (SCFAs). These compounds are renowned for their potent anti-inflammatory effects, helping to regulate immune responses and shield the body from inflammatory conditions. High-fiber foods support a healthy gut microbiome and contribute to the overall inflammation reduction in the body. Integrating fiber-rich foods into your diet is a simple yet effective way to manage inflammation.

Boosting gut health and fortifying your anti-inflammatory eating habits make integrating diverse gut-supportive foods into your daily meals necessary. Excellent sources of probiotics are fermented foods like yogurt and kefir. These foods are often enjoyed on their own or can be blended into smoothies for a nutritious snack. Other fermented foods, including sauerkraut and kimchi, also contribute beneficial bacteria along with an array of nutrients. High-fiber vegetables such as broccoli, Brussels sprouts, and carrots provide the foundation for healthy gut bacteria and are packed with antioxidants and other nutrients that further support inflammation management.

By understanding the vital relationship between gut health and inflammation, you can take proactive steps to nurture your gut microbiome with the right foods. The right foods help maintain your gut health and have far-reaching effects on your overall inflammatory status, immunity, and well-being. Remember, a healthy gut is your friend in the fight against inflammation, and nurturing it with the proper diet can significantly improve your health.

Balancing Macronutrients for Optimal Health

Understanding the roles and balancing the intake of macronutrients —carbohydrates, proteins, and fats—is foundational to managing inflammation effectively. Each macronutrient plays a specific role in keeping your body healthy. Carbohydrates are your body's primary energy source, proteins are crucial for building and repairing tissues, and fats provide a concentrated source of energy as well as aiding in the absorption of vitamins. However, not all macronutrients are created equal, especially in the context of an anti-inflammatory diet. The quality and the ratio in which you consume these nutrients can significantly influence inflammation levels in your body.

The ideal ratios of macronutrients can vary based on individual health needs. However, a general guideline for an anti-inflammatory diet emphasizes a higher intake of healthy fats and proteins with moderate consumption of carbohydrates, primarily from whole, unprocessed sources. It's critical to focus on the quality of macronutrients. For example, complex carbohydrates like whole grains, known to have a lower glycemic index and higher fiber content, help to regulate blood sugar levels and reduce inflammatory responses. Similarly, integrating high-quality proteins and healthy fats into your diet can help manage inflammation more effectively.

Protein plays a pivotal role in managing inflammation and supporting tissue repair. Ensuring you consume enough protein is vital for producing the new proteins essential to your body's healing process, particularly for repairing tissues affected by inflammation. The source of protein is important. Lean proteins like chicken, fish, and turkey, as well as plant-based options like legumes and quinoa, are preferable. These sources provide the necessary amino acids for healing without the excessive saturated fats found in some cuts of red meat. Including a wide variety of protein sources ensures a broader range of nutrients that, in turn, help maintain muscle mass, which is considered essential for overall health.

Fats are perhaps the most misunderstood macronutrients and are often vilified in diet culture. Yet, fats are essential, especially for their role in inflammation. Healthy fats, like those found in avocados, nuts, seeds, and olive oil, provide omega-3 fatty acids known for their anti-inflammatory properties. These fats help produce hormones that regulate inflammation and maintain the structure of every cell in your body. On the other hand, unhealthy fats, including trans fats and certain saturated fats, can trigger inflammatory responses. These are typically found in fried foods, certain baked goods, and processed snack foods. Selecting healthier fats over harmful ones plays a crucial role in moderating your body's inflammation.

Incorporating the proper balance of macronutrients into your diet isn't just about reducing inflammation. It's also about building a sustainable, enjoyable eating pattern that supports your overall health. This eating pattern involves making informed choices about the sources of your macronutrients and understanding how they interact with your body to either promote health or contribute to disease. For instance, replacing some carbohydrate calories with high-quality proteins and fats can help manage blood sugar levels and reduce the risk of type 2 diabetes, a condition closely linked to chronic inflammation. Another strategic choice is opting for whole grains or vegetable-sourced carbohydrates instead of refined grains. This preference aids in preventing the abrupt increases in blood sugar and insulin levels that intensify inflammatory reactions.

Emphasizing the quality over quantity of macronutrients encourages not just a focus on what is eliminated but on what is beneficially included. This approach ensures your meals are nourishing and enjoyable, providing the necessary nutrients to combat inflammation and support your body's overall health. As you adapt to this way of eating, you'll likely notice improvements in how you feel and your overall health outcomes, underlining the profound impact that diet can have on inflammation and wellness.

As we wrap up this exploration of macronutrients and their impact on inflammation, remember that your diet is a powerful tool at your disposal. Modifying your intake of carbohydrates, proteins, and fats to suit your body's needs can help you manage inflammation effectively, leading to better health and an improved quality of life. This holistic approach to nutrition addresses the symptoms associated with inflammation and contributes to lasting wellness. As we move forward, we'll delve deeper into specific dietary strategies and how to implement them in everyday life, ensuring you have the practical knowledge to make the anti-inflammatory diet a seamless part of your routine.

Practical Meal Planning and Preparation

Embarking on an anti-inflammatory diet is about choosing the right foods and weaving these choices into your daily life naturally and sustainably. This chapter is dedicated to transforming these healthy choices into a structured plan that fits seamlessly into your busy schedule, ensuring that maintaining an anti-inflammatory diet is as stress-free as possible. Here, you'll learn how to set realistic meal planning goals, incorporate various anti-inflammatory foods into your weekly routine, and customize these plans to meet your unique dietary needs and preferences.

Designing Your Anti-Inflammatory Meal Plan

Creating a meal plan isn't just about listing what you'll eat for each meal; it's about crafting a strategy that aligns with your health goals, dietary preferences, and lifestyle demands. This structured approach helps in managing inflammation through diet and alleviates the stress of last-minute meal decisions, making healthy eating a practical part of your daily routine.

Setting Realistic Goals

The first step in the meal planning process is setting realistic, achievable goals. Start by assessing your eating habits and identifying areas in which to incorporate more anti-inflammatory foods. The key is to set goals that are ambitious enough to foster positive change but realistic enough to be sustainable. For instance, if you rarely eat vegetables, a goal to include a vegetable with every meal might feel overwhelming. Instead, start by aiming to include vegetables in your dinners. As this becomes a habit, you can gradually expand it to other meals. Remember, the ultimate goal is to make these changes a permanent part of your lifestyle, not just a temporary diet.

Weekly Meal Planning

Planning your meals for the week is one of the most effective ways to ensure you stick to your anti-inflammatory diet. This process involves selecting recipes for each meal and snack for the upcoming week and then shopping for all the ingredients in one go. Begin by choosing recipes that include a variety of anti-inflammatory foods, such as leafy greens, fatty fish, whole grains, and nuts. Plan for meals that are both nourishing and appealing to ensure that your diet remains enjoyable and satisfying.

An effective way to organize this process is to create a meal calendar that outlines what you'll eat for each meal throughout the week. This visual plan helps manage your grocery shopping and takes the guesswork out of meal times, making dietary decisions easier during a busy week. Be sure to include some flexibility in your meal plan for nights when cooking isn't feasible, whether that means planning for leftovers or incorporating a healthy takeout option.

Customization Tips

An essential aspect of successful meal planning is customization. Dietary needs and preferences vary widely, and a one-size-fits-all approach is often not sustainable. If you have particular dietary restrictions or preferences, such as gluten intolerance or vegetarianism, incorporate suitable substitutions into your meals. For instance, if a meal plan suggests grilled salmon, but you're a vegetarian, you could substitute with tofu or a hearty vegetable curry rich in anti-inflammatory spices.

Moreover, aligning your meal plans with your daily life is crucial. For those with a busy schedule, selecting recipes that are quick to prepare or that can be made ahead of time ensures that your plan is realistic and manageable. Tailoring your meal strategy to fit your unique needs and lifestyle increases your chances of success, making it easier to maintain your anti-inflammatory diet amid a hectic life.

Sample Meal Plans

To help you get started, here are a few sample meal plans tailored to an anti-inflammatory diet. Each plan includes a variety of foods to ensure balanced nutrition and broad exposure to different anti-inflammatory compounds:

Day 1

- **Breakfast:** Oatmeal topped with mixed berries and a sprinkle of flaxseeds
- **Lunch:** Grilled chicken salad with mixed greens, cherry tomatoes, avocado, and vinaigrette
- **Dinner:** Baked salmon with quinoa and steamed broccoli
- **Snack:** An apple and a handful of almonds

Day 2

- **Breakfast:** Greek yogurt with honey and walnut pieces
- **Lunch:** Turkey and hummus wrap with spinach and bell peppers
- **Dinner:** Stir-fried tofu with mixed vegetables and a side of brown rice
- **Snack:** Carrot sticks with guacamole

Each meal plan is designed to provide a balanced intake of macronutrients while focusing on anti-inflammatory ingredients. To make these plans work for you, you may adjust the portion sizes and ingredients based on your particular nutritional needs and preferences. Remember, the goal is to make the diet work for you, not to force yourself to adhere to a rigid set of rules.

Grocery Shopping Made Simple: A Buyer's Guide

Navigating the grocery store doesn't have to feel like a chore. With a little preparation and know-how, you can turn your shopping trips into an efficient and enjoyable part of your week. By creating focused shopping lists and understanding how to interpret health claims and seasonal buying options, you can streamline your shopping experience to ensure that it supports your anti-inflammatory diet without stretching your budget or your schedule.

Efficient Shopping Lists

One of the most effective tools at your disposal is the shopping list. A practical list is more than just a reminder of what to buy—it's a strategy that aligns with your meal plans and helps you avoid the common pitfall of impulse purchases, which can often be less healthy options. Start by reviewing your meal plan for the week, and list all the ingredients you will need for each meal. Organize your list by categories based on the layout of your store (e.g., produce, dairy, meats, pantry staples). This approach saves time and helps prevent the back-and-forth when items are forgotten.

A well-organized list also helps you resist the temptation of promotional items that stores often display to encourage impulse buying. With a list in hand, you're more likely to stick to your planned purchases, which support both your health goals and your budget. If you shop for groceries online, many platforms allow you to save your list, making it even easier to reorder staples each week.

Decoding Health Claims

Understanding health claims on packaging is crucial for making informed choices that align with your anti-inflammatory goals. Labels like "natural," "organic," "low-fat," or "reduces cholesterol" can be confusing and sometimes misleading. For example, a "low-fat" label doesn't necessarily mean the product is healthy; it could be high in sugars or artificial additives that are just as detrimental.

When scanning products for health claims, prioritize the nutritional content and ingredient list over the enticing marketing terms. Opt for items with fewer ingredients, which typically suggests minimal processing and additives. Since ingredients are listed in order of proportion within the product, be wary of those with sugars or unfamiliar components leading the list. This careful assessment ensures that each item aligns with your anti-inflammatory diet objectives.

Seasonal Shopping

Shopping for seasonal produce can significantly enhance the quality and effectiveness of your anti-inflammatory diet. Fruits and vegetables are at their nutritional peak when they are in season. They are also more abundant, which can make them less expensive than off-season items shipped from far away. For example, berries are a great source of anti-inflammatory antioxidants, but they can be pricey in the winter when they're not in season. Buying them in the summer when they're locally available can provide you with better nutritional content at a lower cost.

To make the most of seasonal shopping, familiarize yourself with the produce that's in season in your area. Seasonal shopping may mean enjoying hearty root vegetables and squashes in autumn and winter, asparagus and strawberries in the spring, and fruits and vegetables like tomatoes, cucumbers, and peppers in the summer. This strategy bolsters your well-being and budget and introduces a dynamic array of foods into your yearly meal planning, infusing your diet with delightful and intriguing variety.

Local and Organic Options

Exploring local and organic food options is another way to enhance your anti-inflammatory diet. Local foods are often fresher because they don't require long transport times, which can degrade their nutritional quality. Buying local also supports your community's economy and lowers the environmental impact of transporting foods over long distances.

Organic foods, while sometimes more expensive, are grown without artificial pesticides and fertilizers, which can be beneficial if you're trying to reduce your exposure to potentially harmful chemicals that can contribute to inflammation. When shopping for organic foods, prioritize food items known to have higher pesticide residues when grown conventionally. These food items are often called the "dirty dozen" and include strawberries, spinach, grapes, cherries, tomatoes, and apples, among others.

Combining local and organic shopping can maximize the nutritional benefits of your purchases while supporting sustainable practices. Many farmers' markets offer organic produce, providing an excellent opportunity to buy the freshest seasonal items while contributing to local agriculture. Remember, the closer you get to the source of your food, the more control you have over what goes into your body, and the more you can ensure that your dietary choices help reduce inflammation.

Prepping Meals in Advance: Time-Saving Tips

One of the most effective strategies for maintaining a consistent anti-inflammatory diet, especially for those with a busy schedule, is to prepare meals in advance. This approach saves time during your hectic weekdays and helps you adhere to your dietary goals by having healthy, ready-to-eat meals at your disposal. Let's explore some fundamental techniques and tools that can streamline your meal preparation process, making it easier and more efficient.

Batch Cooking Fundamentals

Batch cooking means that you cook larger quantities of food at once. The food can then be stored and used throughout the week. This practice is especially useful for staples like grains, proteins, and vegetables that can be combined and matched to create different meals. For example, you could roast a large tray of mixed vegetables, cook a big pot of quinoa, and grill several chicken breasts simultaneously. Throughout the week, these can be combined in different ways to create meals like salads, wraps, or bowls with minimal additional preparation time.

The key to successful batch cooking is planning. Start by choosing recipes that are versatile and can be easily stored. Make sure you have enough variety to keep your meals interesting throughout the week. You could cook two or three main proteins, a variety of vegetables, and a couple of different whole grains. Once prepared, you can refrigerate these batches and easily combine them into diverse and appealing meals throughout the week.

Storage and Preservation

Appropriate storage is crucial to preserving the freshness and nutritional value of your prepped meals. Use airtight containers to store your cooked foods in the refrigerator or freezer. Glass containers are ideal as they don't harbor bacteria or odors and can be used in both the microwave and the oven for easy reheating. Labeling your containers with the contents and date helps keep track of what you have and ensures minimal waste.

When freezing, cool your foods entirely before transferring them to the freezer. By cooling the foods, you avoid the formation of ice crystals and, in turn, help maintain the quality and texture of the food. Divide meals into single-serving portions for easy thawing and reheating. Remember, freezing can significantly extend the shelf life of your meals, making it an excellent option for those who like to cook in bulk but worry about food spoiling.

Efficient Kitchen Tools

Investing in the right kitchen tools can dramatically reduce the time you spend preparing meals. A good chef's knife and a large cutting board can make chopping vegetables and meats much quicker and easier. Using slow cookers and pressure cookers are excellent ways to make soups, stews, and tender meats with minimal hands-on time. You may also use a blender or food processor for sauces, smoothies, or chopping vegetables.

Another handy tool is a mandoline slicer, which can quickly slice or julienne vegetables in uniform sizes, perfect for salads or stir-fries. When roasting or baking, silicone baking mats and parchment paper are great for easy cleanup. Having these tools at your disposal can streamline your meal preparation process, making it faster and more enjoyable.

Time-Saving Cooking Techniques

Besides batch cooking, you can use several other techniques to save time in the kitchen. One-pan meals are a fantastic way to reduce both cooking and cleaning time. Recipes that use a single skillet, pot, or sheet pan can be nutritious and flavorful with very little cleanup required. Examples include sheet-pan roasted chicken and vegetables, one-pot whole-wheat penne pasta with spinach and red bell peppers, or a skillet stir-fry which could include ingredients like shrimp, red bell peppers and broccoli.

Harnessing the power of a pressure cooker can be a game-changer for those looking to save time. This method allows you to prepare meals in a fraction of the time it would typically take. Ideal for quickly whipping up stews, curries, and grains such as rice and quinoa, pressure cookers enable you to prepare large quantities of staples efficiently. This practice makes it easier to incorporate a variety of healthy, anti-inflammatory dishes into your weekly meal plan. Modern pressure cookers can cook meals in a fraction of the time it takes to cook them traditionally.

Using pre-cut vegetables can also cut down on prep time. Many grocery stores offer fresh or frozen chopped vegetables that are ready to cook. While they may be more expensive than whole vegetables, during particularly busy periods, the time they save may be worth the cost.

Adopting these meal-prepping strategies ensures that maintaining an anti-inflammatory diet doesn't feel like a burden, even on your busiest days. Batch cooking, efficient storage, and the use of helpful kitchen tools can transform meal preparation from a chore into a simple, manageable part of your weekly routine. With these systems in place, you'll find it much easier to eat healthily and reduce inflammation, allowing you more time to enjoy the other important aspects of your life.

Quick and Easy Anti-Inflammatory Breakfast Ideas

Starting your day with a proper breakfast can set the tone for a nourishing day, especially when managing chronic inflammation. A morning meal that combines good sources of protein, fats, and carbohydrates can stabilize blood sugar levels, fuel your morning activities, and keep inflammation at bay. Let's explore some practical, tasty, quick breakfast ideas that align with your anti-inflammatory diet and fit seamlessly into your busy lifestyle.

Breakfasts in Minutes

For many, mornings are rushed, but that doesn't mean you have to skip a nutritious breakfast.

- **Smoothies are an excellent option for a quick and healthy start.** They can be packed with anti-inflammatory ingredients such as spinach, kale, berries, and avocado, blended with a protein source like Greek yogurt or a scoop of protein powder. Add a tablespoon of chia seeds or flaxseeds to boost your intake of omega-3 fatty acids, which are excellent for combating inflammation. The beauty of smoothies lies in their versatility and speed—toss the ingredients into a blender, and you have a portable, incredibly healthy breakfast within minutes.
- **Overnight oats are another excellent choice for those with little time in the mornings.** Before going to bed, mix rolled oats with almond milk or another plant-based milk, a pinch of cinnamon, and your choice of anti-inflammatory fruits like berries or diced apples. Let this sit in the fridge overnight, and by morning, you'll have a creamy, delicious breakfast waiting for you. This dish saves time and provides a good balance of complex carbohydrates and fiber, which are ideal for long-lasting energy and maintaining good digestive health.
- **Egg dishes such as scrambles or omelets can also be made quickly.** Eggs are a fantastic source of high-quality protein and nutrients like vitamins D and B, which are essential for immune function and energy metabolism.

Sauté some spinach, tomatoes, and mushrooms in olive oil—another anti-inflammatory powerhouse—then add your eggs to make an omelet. This meal can be prepared in under ten minutes, providing a savory, satisfying start to your day.

On-the-Go Options

Having on-the-go options ready is essential for those mornings when you're really pressed for time.

- **Homemade granola bars are an excellent choice.** You can make them in advance using oats, nuts, seeds, and some honey or maple syrup to bind them together. Add anti-inflammatory spices like turmeric or ginger for an extra health boost. These bars are not only portable but also packed with nutrients that support sustained energy and help manage inflammation.
- **Another quick, portable breakfast option is fruit-nut combos.** Pair a banana or an apple with a small handful of walnuts or almonds. The fruits provide a fast source of energy and antioxidants. At the same time, the nuts offer satisfying protein and healthy fats, making this a balanced, mobile snack that can curb hunger and provide the necessary fuel until your next meal.

Make-Ahead Solutions

For those who like to plan ahead, make-ahead breakfast recipes can be a lifesaver during a busy week.

- **Breakfast casseroles**: For this option, you can layer vegetables, potatoes, eggs, and perhaps some lean turkey bacon in a baking dish to cook in the oven. Once baked, you can refrigerate portions and simply reheat them in the morning. This option streamlines your morning routine and ensures you have a hearty, inflammation-fighting meal to start your day.
- **Breakfast muffins**: Made with almond flour, bananas, blueberries, and a touch of honey, these can be baked ahead of time and stored. These muffins are not only delicious but also packed with nutrients that support an anti-inflammatory diet. They're easy to grab on your way out the door and can be enjoyed without interrupting your busy morning workflow.

Balancing Macronutrients

Each breakfast option must include a good balance of proteins, fats, and carbohydrates. This balance helps manage blood sugar levels, which is critical for controlling inflammation. A breakfast that includes Greek yogurt (protein) mixed with nuts (fats) and berries (carbohydrates) is an example of a meal that is not only quick to prepare but also gives you a well-rounded start to the day. Ensuring that each meal has this balance will help bolster your energy levels throughout the morning and keep inflammation in check.

Including these quick, nutritious, and versatile breakfast options into your routine makes adhering to an anti-inflammatory diet feasible and enjoyable. These meals provide the nutrients needed to combat inflammation while also catering to your busy schedule, proving that a healthy diet can indeed fit into a fast-paced lifestyle. Remember, the key to a sustainable diet is simplicity and preparation; with these breakfast ideas, you're well-equipped to start each day with both.

Lunches to Reduce Flare-Ups While at Work

Maintaining an anti-inflammatory diet during a hectic workday can be challenging, especially when surrounded by convenient but potentially harmful food choices. Preparing and packing your lunch helps you control your intake of anti-inflammatory foods and ensures you're fueled and focused throughout the day. Here, we delve into the art of packing nutritious, appealing lunches that align with your dietary goals and help you manage inflammation effectively.

Packing Anti-Inflammatory Lunches

The key to a successful anti-inflammatory lunch is balance and preparation. Start by choosing ingredients that are rich in nutrients and known for their anti-inflammatory properties. A balanced lunch should include a good mix of lean protein, fibrous carbohydrates, healthy fats, and plenty of vegetables. For protein, consider grilled chicken or baked salmon. If you prefer a plant-based option, consider legumes like chickpeas and lentils. Combine these with colorful vegetables such as spinach, bell peppers, and carrots. Add complex carbohydrates like quinoa or sweet potatoes, which provide sustained energy without spiking your blood sugar levels.

When assembling your lunch, think about how it will hold up until you're ready to eat. Use airtight containers to keep your food fresh and separate components like dressings or toppings that might make your meal soggy if they sit too long. If you're short on time in the mornings, consider preparing your lunches the night before. The preparation can involve simple tasks like washing and chopping vegetables, cooking grains, or portioning out your proteins. Having these steps completed beforehand makes assembling your lunch quick and efficient. Adopting this approach to meal preparation can lighten your morning routine, affording you some time to relax before your day begins.

Salad Mastery

Salads are a staple for healthy lunches because they are versatile and can be very nutritious. However, nobody enjoys a soggy salad come lunchtime. To master the art of the lunch salad, start with a base of wholesome greens like kale or spinach, which tend to hold up better than softer varieties like lettuce. Add a variety of other vegetables, fresh or roasted, for texture and flavor. For proteins, grilled chicken, hard-boiled eggs, or a scoop of quinoa can make your salad more filling and satisfying.

Placing your salad dressing in a separate package is the key to a great salad that doesn't wilt by lunchtime. Small containers or even reused spice jars are perfect for this. Additionally, layer your ingredients strategically. Place heavier items like proteins and grains at the bottom and lighter, more delicate items like greens and fresh herbs at the top. When lunchtime arrives, effortlessly mix your ingredients to enjoy a salad that's as crisp and fresh as if you just prepared it. This approach guarantees your meal meets your anti-inflammatory dietary objectives and delights your palate.

Thermos-Friendly Foods

Hot lunches can be a comforting midday treat, especially during the colder months. Foods suitable for a thermos offer the comfort of a warm meal that retains its flavor and texture, making them an ideal choice for your midday nourishment. The melding of flavors over time can lead to a more enriched and satisfying meal experience.

- Soups and stews packed with anti-inflammatory ingredients like turmeric, ginger, and garlic are perfect for this. Make a large batch at the beginning of the week, and you'll have a quick, easy lunch option that just needs reheating in the morning before pouring it into your thermos.
- Chili is another great option. A bean-based chili with plenty of spices, tomatoes, and lean ground turkey can be a hearty, inflammation-fighting lunch. The key to a good thermos meal is making sure it's heated thoroughly in the morning; this ensures it stays warm until lunchtime and helps maintain the taste and safety of the food.

Snacks for Sustained Energy

Maintaining energy levels throughout the workday is crucial, and healthy snacks can play a significant role. Select snacks that are easy to prepare and carry, and that will help sustain your energy levels without causing inflammation.

- Mixed nuts, rich in omega-3 fatty acids, are an excellent choice. They're easy to pack and provide a good mix of protein, fat, and fiber that can help tide you over until your next meal.

- Other great options include Greek yogurt with a handful of berries or sliced cucumber with hummus.

Both are simple to prepare and provide a good combination of macronutrients to keep you feeling full and energized. Packing these snacks in small containers or bags makes them easy to grab from your desk or break room. They can help you avoid reaching for less healthy, inflammatory options when hunger strikes between meals.

By adding these strategies into your daily routine, you can ensure that your lunch satisfies your taste buds and supports your health goals. Whether you are enjoying a vibrant, crisp salad or a warm, soothing soup, your lunch can be a powerful tool in your journey to reduce inflammation and maintain your well-being, even on the busiest days.

Simple and Satisfying Anti-Inflammatory Dinners

Dinner is more than just a meal. It's a chance to unwind after a long day and spend quality time with family or enjoy a moment of solitude with a nourishing meal. Creating dinners that adhere to anti-inflammatory guidelines while also catering to the tastes of everyone at the table can seem challenging. However, with a few creative strategies and recipes, it's entirely possible to please both the palate and your health needs.

Family-Friendly Dinners

When preparing meals that need to appeal to all family members, including children, it's essential to incorporate familiar flavors and dishes with a twist of anti-inflammatory ingredients.

- Classic spaghetti and meatballs can be transformed by using whole grain or legume-based pasta paired with turkey meatballs that include herbs like oregano and an anti-inflammatory powerhouse like garlic. Toss in a rich tomato sauce simmered with olive oil and more spices, and you have a comforting, familiar dish that everyone will love but with added health benefits.
- Another family favorite, tacos, can be made anti-inflammatory by using lean proteins like fish or chicken, topped with avocado slices, a squeeze of lime, and a slaw made from red cabbage, carrots, and a hint of apple cider vinegar and honey dressing.

These meals are nutritious and packed with flavors that appeal to various taste preferences, ensuring everyone leaves the table satisfied.

Quick Dinner Fixes

Having a repertoire of quick, anti-inflammatory dinners can be a lifesaver on those hectic weeknights when time is scarce.

- Stir-frying is a rapid cooking method that can feature a mix of protein and a variety of vegetables. For an anti-inflammatory stir-fry, use ingredients like broccoli, bell peppers, and snap peas, and toss them with a protein like shrimp or tofu in a sauce made with ginger, turmeric, and a splash of low-sodium soy sauce or tamari. Serve this over a bed of brown rice or quinoa for a complete meal in less than thirty minutes.
- Another quick option is to whip up a hearty soup using pre-chopped veggies, low-sodium vegetable broth, and

chunks of chicken or beans—season with herbs and spices instead of salt to boost the anti-inflammatory properties and flavor.

Cooking for One or Two

Cooking for fewer people doesn't mean you have to give up on variety or eat leftovers for days. Instead, it offers the flexibility to experiment with dishes without worrying about large quantities.

One practical approach is to prepare one or two larger batches of versatile ingredients at the start of the week, such as roasted vegetables and grilled chicken breast. These can then be used to create different meals throughout the week. For example, one night could be a chicken salad with mixed greens, nuts, and a vinaigrette, and another night could feature a vegetable stir-fry with slices of grilled chicken. Make use of a variety of spices and herbs to transform these staples into entirely different meals, keeping your diet exciting and flavorful.

Integrating Global Flavors

One delightful way to enhance the anti-inflammatory diet is to draw inspiration from global cuisines, which often use spices and herbs extensively. Indian cuisine, for example, offers turmeric and ginger, both known for their potent anti-inflammatory effects. A simple curry dish using these spices, along with coconut milk and a heap of vegetables, can provide a warming, therapeutic meal.

Similarly, you can bring Mediterranean flavors into your kitchen with dishes like Greek lemon chicken with oregano, garlic, and olives, served alongside a salad tossed with extra virgin olive oil and plenty of fresh herbs. By exploring these global flavors, you broaden your culinary horizons and also enhance the anti-inflammatory potential of your meals.

Applying these strategies to your dinner routines ensures that your meals are not only nutritious and aligned with your health goals but also diverse and enjoyable. Whether you're cooking for a family, making a quick meal after a long day, or preparing a quiet dinner for one, these ideas can help maintain variety in your diet and make every dinner a delightful, health-promoting experience.

As this chapter on practical meal planning and preparation concludes, remember that the key to successfully managing an anti-inflammatory diet is thoughtful preparation, creative cooking, and enjoying the process. Each meal is an opportunity to nourish your body and delight your senses, providing both the nutrients needed to combat inflammation and the pleasure that makes eating such a fundamental joy of life. As you move forward, carry these strategies and tips with you into the next chapter of your journey toward a healthier, more vibrant life.

Delicious Recipes That Won't Break the Bank

Eating healthily often carries a stigma of high expense and exclusivity, particularly when aiming to adhere to an anti-inflammatory diet. However, this chapter will guide you through the maze of budget-friendly options that do not compromise quality or flavor. Here, you'll discover how to enjoy nutritious, anti-inflammatory meals without stretching your finances. Let's dive into a world where health meets cost-efficiency, making it possible for anyone, regardless of budget, to embrace a lifestyle that combats inflammation and promotes wellness, all without breaking the bank.

Budget-Friendly Anti-Inflammatory Ingredients

Identifying Cost-Effective Ingredients

A cornerstone of maintaining an affordable anti-inflammatory diet is knowing which ingredients offer the best value for money while providing significant health benefits. Staples such as lentils, beans, bulk whole grains, and seasonal vegetables cost less than many processed foods and are rich in nutrients that help fight inflammation. Lentils and beans, for example, are not just affordable but also incredibly versatile. Lentils and beans are considered excellent sources of protein and fiber, which help reduce inflammation markers in the body. Beans, including lentils, can be used in various dishes, such as soups, stews, salads, and side dishes, allowing you to get creative with your meals. Whole grains, such as brown rice, barley, and oats, offer high fiber content, which is essential for gut health. They play a crucial role in managing body-wide inflammation. By focusing on these staples, you can build a multitude of meals that are both cost-effective and anti-inflammatory.

Bulk Buying Tips

Buying ingredients in bulk is a smart strategy that can lead to significant savings and ensure that you always have key anti-inflammatory ingredients on hand. This approach saves you money and reduces the frequency of shopping trips, making it easier to stick to your healthy eating plan.

Items like nuts, seeds, and spices are typically cheaper when bought in bulk. However, to maintain their freshness and nutritional value, nuts and seeds should be kept in airtight containers in a cool, dark place to prevent them from becoming rancid. Spices, while having a longer shelf life, should also be stored away from heat and light to preserve their potent anti-inflammatory properties.

Seasonal Shopping Strategies

Embracing seasonal shopping is a powerful strategy to enhance the affordability of your anti-inflammatory diet. Fruits and vegetables bought in season are often cheaper and richer in nutrients than those that are out of season and have been transported long distances. By selecting fruits and vegetables that are at their nutritional peak, you can cut costs and boost nutrition. These timely picks contribute to meal variety and flavor, all while delivering potent anti-inflammatory advantages.

Simple Swaps for Expensive Items

Adopting an anti-inflammatory diet doesn't mean you have to splurge on expensive superfoods or supplements. Simple swaps can help you maintain the diet without overspending. For example, instead of purchasing costly supplements, use herbs and spices like turmeric and ginger to flavor your meals and gain anti-inflammatory benefits. Similarly, opt for olive oil, a staple of the anti-inflammatory diet, instead of more exotic oils that can be pricier. This strategy ensures your meals are affordable and emphasizes the consumption of whole-food sources of anti-inflammatory nutrients, which are often more effectively absorbed by the body than their supplement counterparts.

Focusing on these budget-friendly strategies and ingredients can help you manage inflammation effectively through your diet without financial strain. This approach supports your physical health and ensures that your healthy eating habits are sustainable and enjoyable, free from the stress of high grocery bills. As you continue to explore these strategies, remember that every meal is a chance to nourish your body and contribute to your long-term well-being, all while being mindful of your budget.

Family-Friendly Recipes Everyone Will Love

Creating meals that cater to the tastes of both children and adults while sticking to the principles of an anti-inflammatory diet might seem challenging. However, it's a delightful journey that's entirely achievable with a bit of creativity and planning. One of the joys of cooking family-friendly meals is the opportunity to prepare dishes that are as enjoyable to eat as they are healthy. Smoothies, homemade pizzas with whole grain crusts, and veggie-packed pasta dishes are just a few examples that can be adapted to suit everyone's taste buds and dietary needs.

- **Smoothies**: These are a fantastic way to incorporate a variety of anti-inflammatory ingredients in a form that's usually more acceptable to kids. Blend fruits such as berries, which are rich in antioxidants, with vegetables like spinach or kale that might otherwise be a hard sell on their own. Add a base of almond milk or Greek yogurt for a creamy texture, a boost of protein, and maybe a spoonful of chia seeds or flaxseeds to elevate the omega-3 fatty acid content. This type of meal provides essential nutrients and comes in a familiar, often beloved form. Even better, smoothies are quick to prepare, making them ideal for busy mornings or as a nutritious snack.
- **Homemade pizzas**: Another versatile option. By using whole grain crusts, you increase the fiber content, which is beneficial for maintaining a healthy gut—a critical factor in managing inflammation. Top these pizzas with tomato sauce rich in lycopene, an anti-inflammatory compound, and a selection of toppings like grilled chicken, arugula, bell peppers, and a sprinkle of mozzarella cheese. Allowing children to participate in meal preparation, particularly

with homemade pizzas, transforms the experience into an interactive activity. Children become part of the culinary process by selecting and topping their pizzas with a wide variety of healthy ingredients. These activities make mealtime more delightful and encourage a more profound commitment to nutritious eating.

- **Veggie-packed pasta dishes**: These are also a hit. Choose whole-grain or legume-based pasta as a healthier alternative to traditional white pasta. Sauté a mix of vegetables like zucchini, cherry tomatoes, and spinach in olive oil—a healthy fat known for its anti-inflammatory properties—and toss them with the pasta. A light sauce made from puréed roasted red peppers or butternut squash can add flavor and creaminess without the need for heavy creams or cheeses. This meal is not only filling and nutritious but also colorful and appealing to children, making it easier to introduce them to a wide variety of vegetables in an enticing way.
- **Children**: Bringing children into the kitchen to help with meal preparation can significantly alter their perspective on food and health. Assigning simple kitchen tasks like mixing ingredients, rinsing vegetables, or setting the dinner table imparts a sense of responsibility and accomplishment. Moreover, this collaborative effort in meal preparation strengthens family bonds, creating lasting memories associated with good nutrition and healthy lifestyle choices. It helps them understand where their food comes from and what goes into preparing it, fostering a deeper appreciation for eating healthily. Simple tasks like stirring the batter, washing vegetables, or setting the table give them a sense of responsibility and achievement. Cooking together can be a bonding activity

that creates fond memories associated with healthy eating habits.

Adjusting meals to suit various tastes without compromising nutritional value is crucial in a family setting. For instance, if some family members prefer small amounts of spice, you can always serve chili flakes or hot sauce on the side rather than cooking them into the dish. Similarly, if textures are an issue, especially for younger children, choose softer-cooked vegetables or chop them finely before adding them to dishes like the pasta mentioned earlier. These minor adjustments ensure that the meals meet everyone's preferences and dietary requirements while maintaining their anti-inflammatory benefits.

Quick and easy meals are essential for any busy family. One-pot dishes save time not only on cooking but also on cleaning. For example, a one-pot chicken and vegetable stew can be a great way to incorporate anti-inflammatory ingredients into a single, hearty dish.

- First, sauté onions and garlic in olive oil. Then, add chicken pieces and a selection of vegetables, such as carrots, potatoes, and celery.
- Pour in a low-sodium chicken broth and simmer until everything is cooked.
- Herbs like rosemary and thyme add flavor and additional anti-inflammatory properties.

Meals like this are straightforward to make. They ensure that dinner is nutritious and keep everyone satisfied and healthy.

These strategies and recipes allow you to successfully incorporate anti-inflammatory eating into your family's routine. These meals prove that health-focused food can be colorful, delicious, and embraced by all ages, making your journey toward a healthier lifestyle a shared, enjoyable family adventure.

Comfort Foods: Healthy Twists on Classic Favorites

Comfort foods are often synonymous with warmth and nostalgia, evoking memories of meals shared with loved ones. However, traditional comfort foods can sometimes be laden with ingredients that stimulate inflammation, such as refined sugars, unhealthy fats, and processed grains. The good news is that you can still indulge in these beloved dishes by tweaking them with healthier, anti-inflammatory alternatives that are just as satisfying and flavorful.

Reinventing Classics

Let's start by reimagining some classic comfort foods. Consider the much-loved French fries—typically deep-fried and salted. Instead of using white potatoes and submerging them in oil, try sweet potatoes cut into wedges, lightly tossed with olive oil and a pinch of sea salt, and baked in the oven. Sweet potatoes are lower on the glycemic index and rich in beta-carotene, an antioxidant that fights inflammation. Another comfort classic is macaroni and cheese, a dish traditionally heavy on dairy and refined pasta. By swapping out regular pasta for one made from quinoa or brown rice and creating a creamy sauce from puréed cashews or a mix of nutritional yeast and almond milk, you maintain the creamy texture and comforting taste without the inflammatory effects of dairy and refined carbs.

Gluten-Free Options

Adapting comfort foods to be gluten-free doesn't mean you'll lose out on taste or texture. Gluten, which is found in wheat, barley, and rye, can be problematic for those with sensitivities or celiac disease and may contribute to inflammation in sensitive individuals. Fortunately, many delicious alternatives align well with anti-inflammatory needs. For instance, pasta dishes can be recreated using gluten-free grains like quinoa or rice. Quinoa pasta mimics the texture of traditional pasta and adds a valuable protein component that's essential for tissue repair and maintenance. Similarly, bread can be made using almond or coconut flour instead of wheat flour. These alternatives provide healthier fats and are lower in carbs, helping manage blood sugar levels and reduce inflammation.

Reducing Unhealthy Fats

The method of cooking can significantly influence the healthiness of comfort food. Traditional frying methods often involve cooking foods in unhealthy fats at high temperatures and can produce inflammation-promoting compounds. An excellent way to enjoy fried foods without the downside is to use an air fryer or oven-baking method. For example, chicken tenders can be coated in an almond flour mixture and baked or air-fried to achieve the same crispy texture without deep-frying. This method significantly reduces the unhealthy fat content while still satisfying that craving for crunchy comfort.

Enhancing Flavors Naturally

The flavor in meals often comes from high-sodium sauces and seasonings, which can be detrimental in large amounts. Instead, enhance the flavor of dishes using natural herbs and spices, many of which offer anti-inflammatory benefits.

For instance, you can add turmeric to soups and stews for a warm, earthy flavor and its excellent anti-inflammatory properties. Herbs like rosemary and thyme add depth to dishes and contain compounds that can help reduce inflammation. By making these adjustments, you can transform comfort foods into a healing, nourishing experience that still brings the joy and satisfaction of traditional favorites.

Through these adaptations, comfort foods can be enjoyed in a way that contributes positively to your health, allowing you to indulge in delicious flavors without compromising your anti-inflammatory lifestyle goals. Whether it's a crispy batch of fries or a creamy bowl of macaroni and cheese, these dishes can be skillfully and healthfully reinvented to provide comfort that nourishes both the body and soul.

Snacks and Small Bites for Busy Days

In the rhythm of your busy day-to-day life, eating the right snacks can be a game-changer, especially when you're aiming to adhere to an anti-inflammatory diet. Snacks are not just about staving off hunger; they're about strategically re-fueling your body throughout the day without causing inflammation. Ideally, they should be easy to prepare, convenient to carry, and delicious enough to look forward to. Here, I'll share some excellent choices that check all these boxes, ensuring you can maintain your health goals even on your busiest days without missing a beat.

- **Homemade trail mix**: One of those wonderful snack options you can customize to suit your taste and health needs. First, choose your base of nuts, which may be almonds, walnuts, or cashews. Nuts are typically rich in omega-3 fatty acids and have been shown to help reduce inflammation. Add some seeds like pumpkin or sunflower for variety and extra nutrients. Enhance the natural sweetness of your trail mix by including dried fruits like cherries or apricots. It's essential to select options that do not have added sugars or preservatives to keep your snack both delicious and anti-inflammatory. A sprinkle of cinnamon or turmeric can boost the anti-inflammatory power of your trail mix while adding a touch of flavor. The beauty of trail mix is that it's not only nutritious but also highly portable. Pack it in small, airtight containers or zip-lock bags, and you have the perfect on-the-go snack that won't spoil quickly.

- **Veggie chips**: These provide another outstanding snack option that's both satisfying and beneficial for your health. You can make a large batch of kale, sweet potato, or beet chips in advance and have them ready for snacking throughout the week. Slice your chosen vegetables thinly. Toss the sliced vegetables with a bit of olive oil, add your preferred herbs or spices, then bake them in the oven until crispy. These chips are lower in calories and fat than regular potato chips and provide valuable nutrients and fiber, essential for maintaining a healthy immune response and reducing inflammation.
- **Hummus with raw vegetables**: A powerhouse snack that combines protein, fiber, and healthy fats. Chickpeas, the main component of hummus, is an excellent source of protein and fiber, while tahini (sesame seed paste) provides a rich supply of anti-inflammatory fats. Pair the hummus with cucumber slices, carrots, or bell peppers for extra

vitamins and antioxidants. This snack is filling and helps keep your energy levels stable, thanks to its balanced combination of macronutrients. Plus, it's easy to pack and stays fresh in a small container, making it an ideal choice for those hectic days when you need a fast and healthy pick-me-up.
- For those times when you need a snack that satisfies your hunger and boosts your energy levels, consider combinations that include proteins and healthy fats. Nut butter with apple slices is a classic example—simple yet effective. The apple provides a quick source of energy from natural sugars and fiber, while the nut butter offers protein and healthy fats that slow the absorption of sugar, preventing spikes in blood sugar levels. Another great option is Greek yogurt topped with berries and a sprinkle of chia seeds. This snack is rich in protein, probiotics, and antioxidants, making it an excellent choice for an energy boost that also supports your digestive and immune health.

Finding snacks that are both healthy for and appealing to children may seem challenging, but it's perfectly achievable with a bit of creativity.

- **Oatmeal bars**: You can bake a batch using oats, mashed bananas for natural sweetness, and add-ins like nuts or berries. Cut these into bars for a snack that kids can enjoy at school or after activities.
- **Fruit and cheese kabobs**: Another fun and healthy option. Alternate pieces of cheese with grapes or chunks of pineapple on skewers for a tasty snack that is fun to eat and packed with nutrients like calcium and vitamins.

Each of these snacks is designed to fit seamlessly into your life, ensuring that you can maintain your anti-inflammatory diet without fuss, no matter how packed your schedule. They provide the nutrition you need to keep inflammation at bay. They are also simple, portable, and enjoyable to eat—perfect for sustaining you through your busy days and contributing to your overall well-being.

Decadent Desserts without the Guilt

Indulging in desserts while maintaining an anti-inflammatory diet might seem like a balancing act. However, with the right ingredients and techniques, you can enjoy sweet treats that are delicious and beneficial to your health. Natural sweeteners, fruit-based recipes, and healthy fats can transform the typical guilt-laden dessert into a wholesome, satisfying finale to any meal.

Sweetening Naturally

Refined sugars are a common culprit behind spikes in inflammation, but that doesn't mean you have to give up on sweetness. Natural sweeteners like honey, maple syrup, and stevia offer the pleasure of sweetness without the inflammatory effects associated with processed sugar. Honey, for instance, not only sweetens your desserts but also brings antioxidants that combat inflammation. Maple syrup, another excellent choice, provides minerals like zinc and manganese, which support immune function and reduce inflammation. Stevia, a plant-based sweetener, contains compounds known as steviol glycosides that have been shown to have anti-inflammatory properties and are calorie-free, making it an excellent option for those managing calorie intake. Using these natural sweeteners allows you to indulge in the rich sweetness of your desserts without triggering the inflammation and health issues associated with refined sugars.

Fruit-Based Desserts

Fruits are nature's candy and a powerful tool in your anti-inflammatory arsenal. They are rich in fiber, vitamins, and antioxidants. Crafting desserts that spotlight fruits elevates their inherent sweetness and amplifies your consumption of ingredients that fight inflammation.

- Baked apples, for instance, include apples stuffed with nuts and spices and a drizzle of honey, which is then baked until tender. This simple dessert captures the essence of comfort food while being entirely healthful.
- Berry compotes are another suitable option. In them, mixed berries are gently simmered with a touch of maple syrup and served over Greek yogurt or whole-grain pancakes.
- For a tropical twist, a fruit salad featuring mangoes, pineapple, and kiwi, sprinkled with fresh mint and a squeeze of lime, can be both refreshing and anti-inflammatory. These fruit-based desserts are easy to prepare and packed with flavors and nutrients that support your health goals.

Healthy Fats in Desserts

Including healthy fats in desserts can enrich their texture and flavor while contributing to their anti-inflammatory properties.

- Avocados blend seamlessly into a chocolate mousse, providing a creamy texture full of heart-healthy fats

without altering the rich chocolate flavor. Simply blend ripe avocados with cocoa powder, a natural sweetener like honey, and a touch of vanilla for a decadent yet healthy dessert.
- Nuts and seeds are another great addition to desserts, not just for their crunch but for their omega-3 fatty acids, which are known to reduce inflammation.
- Almond butter brownies can be made by substituting flour with almond butter, which enhances the nutty flavor and boosts the nutritional profile of your dessert.

Portion Control Tips

Enjoying desserts is as much about satisfaction as it is about moderation. Serving sizes can significantly affect how desserts impact your health and inflammation levels. By focusing on the quality of ingredients and the pleasure of consuming them, you can satisfy your sweet tooth with smaller portions that incorporate all the flavor and none of the guilt. Opt for smaller serving dishes or individual ramekins when crafting your desserts. This approach aids in managing portion sizes while elevating the indulgence and exclusivity of each serving. Further, by fully immersing yourself in the dessert experience—savoring every bite attentively without distractions—you'll find greater satisfaction in smaller quantities, enhancing your enjoyment and adherence to an anti-inflammatory lifestyle.

In this way, desserts are not just the end of a meal but an integral part of a balanced, anti-inflammatory diet. They provide an opportunity to satisfy cravings creatively and healthily, proving that you can enjoy the sweeter things in life without compromise. With these strategies, desserts transition from indulgent treats to expressions of culinary creativity that support your health and delight your palate.

Celebratory Meals and Special Occasions

Sticking to an anti-inflammatory diet can feel like a challenge when special occasions roll around, from holiday gatherings to family celebrations. However, with thoughtful planning and a few creative strategies, you can prepare delightful meals that keep inflammation at bay and ensure everyone at the table enjoys a festive, delicious spread without feeling restricted.

Planning for Holidays and Gatherings

The key to successful holiday meals lies in planning ahead. Start by mapping out a menu that includes a variety of dishes that are designed to be anti-inflammatory. Focus on including plenty of vegetables, lean proteins, and dishes rich in omega-3s and antioxidants.

- For the main course, a roasted turkey or salmon as the centerpiece provides a high-protein main dish with anti-inflammatory benefits. Surround the turkey with side dishes like a colorful salad tossed with vinaigrette, steamed green beans, and a sweet potato mash.
- Opt for a fruit-based dish like a berry tart made with an almond flour crust for dessert. Preparing a list of what you'll need in advance helps you shop efficiently and gives you the peace of mind that you're ready to create a feast that aligns with your dietary goals.

Recipes for Group Settings

One-pot dishes are great for feeding a crowd without spending all day in the kitchen.

- A large pot of Moroccan-inspired chicken stew infused with anti-inflammatory spices like turmeric, ginger, and cinnamon fills the room with enticing aromas. It provides a hearty meal that is easy to serve.
- Similarly, large salads are perfect for gatherings; try a quinoa salad with roasted beets, arugula, and a citrus dressing. It's not only vibrant and tasty but also packed with nutrients that fight inflammation.

These dishes are ideal because they can be made in advance, are easy to scale up for more guests, and require minimal final prep. Thus, you can enjoy the gathering as much as your guests do.

Alcohol Alternatives

Special occasions often call for a toast, but alcoholic beverages can exacerbate inflammation. Instead, offer your guests a variety of appealing non-alcoholic alternatives that are just as festive.

- Infused waters are simple yet elegant; cucumber, mint, or citrus slices added to water enhance the flavor and provide additional antioxidants.
- Herbal teas, served iced or hot, can be a comforting alternative. Varieties like ginger or peppermint are particularly soothing and anti-inflammatory.
- For a celebratory touch, prepare a non-alcoholic sangria with a mix of sparkling water and a variety of chopped

fruits like oranges, apples, and berries, allowing the natural fruit sugars to create a sweet, festive drink.

Making Room for Indulgence

Finally, it's important to balance indulgence with healthy choices during special events. Allow room for small indulgences, such as a piece of dark chocolate or a slice of a favorite dessert. Moderation is key—enjoying a small portion of something you love can make the celebration feel special without causing significant setbacks to your health goals. Encourage guests to fill their plates with the healthy options first, making less room for high-calorie, inflammatory foods. This strategy helps everyone enjoy a bit of what they love while still filling up on the nutritious, anti-inflammatory dishes you've prepared.

By integrating these strategies into your holiday and special occasion planning, you can create joyful, inclusive celebrations that support your health and delight your guests. These gatherings become opportunities to showcase how delicious and satisfying an anti-inflammatory diet can be without feeling like you're missing out on the festivities. As you move forward, each successful event builds your confidence in maintaining your health goals, even during the most indulgent seasons, ensuring you can fully enjoy every special occasion with peace of mind.

In wrapping up this exploration of celebratory meals and special occasions, remember that maintaining an anti-inflammatory diet during these festive and special occasions is not just about dietary restrictions—it's about creatively adapting traditions and making choices that enhance your health and enjoyment of life's celebratory moments. As your journey progresses, these occasions will deepen your insight into food's integral role in fostering wellness and joy. We now move on to our next conversations on sustaining an anti-inflammatory lifestyle year-round, effortlessly integrating nutritious eating into every occasion.

Overcoming Challenges and Handling Setbacks

Embarking on an anti-inflammatory diet is like setting out on a vibrant path lined with the lush greens of spinach and kale, the bright oranges of sweet potatoes, and the deep blues of berries. However, even the most scenic routes have hurdles and occasional stormy weather. The holidays and festive seasons can often feel like a downpour on your parade, tempting you with dishes that stir nostalgia but are laden with inflammatory ingredients. Consider this chapter your umbrella, designed to help you navigate these challenges without straying from your path to wellness.

Staying on Track during the Holidays

The holiday season is synonymous with joy, family gatherings, and, unavoidably, an abundance of food. While these festivities are a source of happiness, they can also present numerous temptations for those committed to an anti-inflammatory diet. Preparation and balance are crucial to maintaining your dietary goals during this merry but challenging time.

Plan Ahead with Menus

Planning is your first line of defense against the dietary challenges that holidays can present. Before any family gathering or holiday event, take the initiative to plan out menus that include anti-inflammatory dishes. The plan doesn't have to overhaul traditional recipes, but you can integrate healthier options everyone can enjoy. For instance, if you're hosting a dinner, ensure that the menu has a variety of dishes rich in vegetables, lean proteins, and healthy fats. If you're not hosting, find out which dishes will be served and offer to take a dish or two that aligns with your dietary needs. This way, you'll ensure you have tasty and healthy options. Also, this approach will reduce last-minute stress and the likelihood of unhealthy choices.

Healthy Holiday Swaps

Holiday traditions frequently shape the festive menu, brimming with hearty gravies, sweet treats, and an overabundance of refined carbs. However, introducing wholesome alternatives to these classic dishes allows you to relish the celebratory meals without worsening inflammation. For example, try cauliflower mash instead of the usual mashed potatoes, which are often made with lots of butter and cream. Cauliflower is rich in antioxidants and can be prepared to have a similar texture and richness as traditional mashed potatoes but with fewer calories and inflammatory fats. Similarly, for dessert, a spiced pumpkin mousse can replace heavy pies. Using coconut milk and a touch of maple syrup can provide the creamy sweetness you crave without a spike in your sugar levels.

Communicating Dietary Needs

Often, navigating holiday meals involves dining at someone else's home, where you will have less control over the menu. In these instances, communication becomes crucial. Before attending any event, it's beneficial to communicate your dietary preferences with your host. Most hosts will appreciate knowing in advance and may adjust their menu or inform you of the options that meet your needs. When addressing your dietary preferences, it's beneficial to highlight the enjoyable options within your diet instead of cataloging excluded items. Propose contributing a dish to the gathering that aligns with your dietary guidelines while being a delightful addition for all guests. This strategy lightens the load for your host while guaranteeing that you have a tasty and suitable option to enjoy.

Indulgence within Limits

The holidays are a time of celebration, and part of that celebration often involves special foods. Completely depriving yourself of these once-a-year treats can make you feel like an outsider and may even dampen your holiday spirit. The trick is to indulge wisely. Choose one or two "worth it" treats and plan when you'll have them. Savor those treats without guilt, then balance them with healthier choices throughout the rest of the holiday. Also, focus on portion control, which can help you enjoy the flavors of the season without overindulging. Fill most of your plate with anti-inflammatory foods, then add a small portion of your chosen indulgence.

Navigating the holiday season on an anti-inflammatory diet may seem daunting. Yet, with strategic planning, open communication, and intentional indulgence, you can fully participate in holiday celebrations without derailing your journey toward improved health.

Remember, the holiday season is just as much about enjoying the company of loved ones as it is about the food. By focusing on the joy of the season and the company around you, you can create new traditions that celebrate health and happiness.

Navigating Social Gatherings and Eating Out

Adopting an anti-inflammatory lifestyle doesn't have to mean missing out on social gatherings or dining experiences. The secret is in making thoughtful decisions and preparing in advance. This approach ensures that your social engagements and eating habits support your health objectives. You certainly don't have to decline every invitation or dine in solitude. Instead, the goal is to become adept at choosing suitable options and handling social settings in a way that keeps your anti-inflammatory eating plan on track.

Choosing the Right Restaurants

Selecting where to dine is pivotal in managing your diet outside the home. Start by identifying restaurants that offer a range of healthy options or are known for their fresh, whole-food-based meals. Many restaurants now cater to health-conscious consumers or those with specific dietary needs, offering delicious dishes that align with anti-inflammatory guidelines. Before you go, make it a habit to check the restaurant's menu online. This practice can help you plan what to order beforehand, avoiding the rush and pressure of deciding on the spot. Look for dishes rich in vegetables, lean proteins, and healthy fats, and be wary of descriptions that indicate the food may be fried or prepared with creamy or sugary sauces. If the menu needs clarification, feel free to call the restaurant to ask about their dishes. You can also inquire about cooking methods or the possibility of customizing a dish while conversing with the restaurant.

What to Order

The type of cuisine you select plays a crucial role in navigating meal options when you are on an anti-inflammatory diet. For example, when dining at an Italian restaurant, choose dishes like grilled fish with steamed vegetables or a fresh salad with olive oil and vinegar dressing instead of creamy pasta. At Mexican restaurants, choose grilled seafood or chicken dishes and request lettuce wraps instead of tortillas. For Asian cuisine, choose stir-fried or steamed dishes with vegetables and lean proteins, and ask for sauces on the side to control the amount. Avoiding or limiting white rice and asking for brown rice or extra vegetables is also advisable. By understanding the typical ingredients and preparation methods of different cuisines, you can make choices that fit your dietary guidelines without feeling deprived.

Handling Social Pressure

Social settings often include expectations to indulge in whatever is being served, leading to awkward situations if you're trying to stick to an anti-inflammatory diet. The key to handling social pressure is confidence and preparation. If you're comfortable, share your health goals with friends or family beforehand so they know your dietary preferences. Such transparency often leads to supportive conversations rather than peer pressure. When offered a dish that doesn't align with your diet, a polite decline with a simple explanation can suffice, such as saying, "It looks delicious, but I'm currently following a specific eating plan for health reasons." Offering to bring a dish to share that meets your dietary needs can also be a great way to contribute and ensure there's something suitable for you to enjoy.

Portable Snacks

Having portable, anti-inflammatory snacks on hand is a strategic way to ensure you always have suitable options available, especially at gatherings where the menu is out of your control. Pack both convenient and satisfying snacks, like almonds, walnuts, carrot sticks with hummus, or fresh fruit. These can curb your hunger and provide the nutrients needed to adhere to your anti-inflammatory diet, reducing the temptation to indulge in less healthy offerings. Such snacks are beneficial for you and can be shared, introducing others to tasty, healthy alternatives.

Staying true to an anti-inflammatory diet during social events and restaurant outings is achievable with thoughtful planning and tactics, although it may initially seem disheartening. By choosing appropriate restaurants, planning your meals, confidently handling social pressures, and keeping healthy snacks on hand, you can enjoy social interactions and dining experiences without compromising your health. These practices empower you to maintain your dietary choices in various social settings, supporting your journey toward a healthier, calmer lifestyle.

Dealing with Cravings and Temptations

Cravings are a natural part of the human experience, particularly when introducing changes to your diet. Understanding why you crave certain foods is essential for managing and redirecting these desires toward choices that support your health goals. Both psychological factors, such as emotional comfort or habit, and physiological factors, such as hormonal imbalances or nutritional deficiencies, can drive cravings. For example, craving sweets can be a response to low blood sugar levels, signaling your body's desire for a quick source of energy. Alternatively, craving salty foods may indicate stress, as stress hormones can deplete the body's natural salts. Recognizing the root cause of your craving is the first step toward addressing it effectively.

When it comes to managing these cravings, substituting unhealthy choices with healthier, anti-inflammatory alternatives is a practical strategy. If you find yourself craving sweets, opt for natural sweeteners like fresh fruits or dark chocolate that is at least 70 percent cocoa. These alternatives provide the sweetness you desire without the high sugar content that can exacerbate inflammation. Try seasoned nuts or seeds for salty cravings—these satisfy the appetite and provide beneficial fats and nutrients that reduce inflammation. By making these swaps, you address your cravings and contribute positively to your dietary goals.

Mindful eating is another powerful tool in managing cravings. This technique involves being fully present during meals, paying close attention to the flavors, textures, and sensations of the meal, and listening to your body's hunger and fullness cues. Before you give in to a craving:

1. Take a moment to pause and assess whether you are hungry or the craving is driven by emotion or habit.
2. If you determine it's hunger, choose a healthy, filling option.
3. If it's emotional, consider other ways to address that emotion, such as taking a walk, speaking to a friend, or engaging in a hobby. This pause can help you make conscious decisions rather than succumbing to impulsive eating, often leading to choices that don't align with your health objectives.

Stress often triggers cravings, as it can disrupt hormonal balance and lead to emotional eating. Managing stress effectively is, therefore, crucial in maintaining an anti-inflammatory diet. Practicing deep breathing, yoga, and regular exercise reduces stress and improves your overall physical health. These actions, in turn, make it less likely that you will seek comfort in food. Establish a routine that includes these activities, which can provide structure and reduce the likelihood of stress-induced cravings. In addition, ensure you are getting adequate sleep, as sleep deprivation can increase cravings and disrupt the hormones that regulate hunger and satiety.

Understanding the underlying causes of your cravings helps you to adopt healthy substitutes. Choosing these alternatives, practicing mindful eating, and managing stress proactively can help you navigate the temptations that could derail your anti-inflammatory diet. Such strategies are about more than resisting what you crave. They're about transforming your approach to eating and wellness, empowering you to make choices that nourish both your body and mind.

How to Modify Your Favorite Recipes

Adapting your cherished recipes to fit an anti-inflammatory diet doesn't have to mean sacrificing flavor or the joy of cooking. It's about making substitutions and tweaks that align with your health goals while keeping the essence of the dish intact. Understanding how to modify your recipes skillfully can transform your dietary habits, making your favorite meals healthier without losing their original appeal.

Ingredient Substitutions

One of the most effective ways to maintain the flavors in your favorite dishes while making them more health-friendly is to use herbs and spices instead of salt for seasoning. High salt intake is often associated with increased inflammation and health issues such as high blood pressure. Herbs like rosemary, thyme, basil, and spices such as turmeric, ginger, and cinnamon enhance the taste and bring anti-inflammatory benefits to dishes. For instance, curcumin, the active component in turmeric, is well-known for its potent anti-inflammatory properties and can transform a simple meal into a health-boosting feast.

Another common substitution is swapping out refined oils for those with healthier fats. Cooking with oils high in polyunsaturated and monounsaturated fats, such as olive oil or avocado oil, instead of butter or margarine, can significantly reduce the intake of unhealthy saturated fats and enhance your meal's overall nutritional profile.

Additionally, in baking, unsweetened applesauce or mashed bananas can replace butter to reduce fat content and add natural sweetness, allowing for a reduction in added sugars as well.

Reducing Sugar in Recipes

Reducing sugar doesn't mean you have to give up on sweet flavors. Natural sweeteners like stevia, which is much sweeter than sugar but with no calories, can be used in place of sugar in recipes ranging from baked goods to sauces and dressings. Stevia can help manage blood sugar levels, contributing to reduced inflammation. When modifying recipes that involve baking, another technique is to use puréed fruits such as apples, dates, or figs. These fruits provide natural sweetness and add fiber, vitamins, and antioxidants, enhancing the nutritional value of your desserts or baked goods.

For instance, in a muffin recipe calling for a cup of sugar, you could use a half cup of unsweetened apple sauce and a quarter teaspoon of stevia instead. This substitution reduces the calorie and sugar content and adds moisture and flavor. Experimenting with the amounts and types of sweeteners may be necessary to achieve the desired taste and texture, but the health benefits are well worth the effort.

Healthier Cooking Methods

How you cook your food can also impact its inflammatory potential. Techniques such as steaming, grilling, and baking are preferable over frying, as they retain more nutrients and require less fat. Steaming vegetables, for example, is one of the best ways to preserve their color, texture, and antioxidants compared to boiling or frying. When grilling or baking, using marinades rich in herbs, spices, and healthy oils enhances flavor while reducing the formation of harmful compounds that can occur at high temperatures.

Recipe Makeovers

Consider the transformation of a classic beef burger into an anti-inflammatory meal. Traditionally, burgers might be served with a white flour bun, fried potatoes, and condiments rich in sugars and unhealthy fats. A makeover version uses lean ground turkey mixed with chopped spinach and spices like garlic and black pepper for the patty, served on a whole-grain bun or a large lettuce leaf. Replace fries with baked sweet potato wedges seasoned with a sprinkle of rosemary and olive oil. For condiments, opt for a homemade guacamole or a yogurt-based sauce. Such substitutions not only reduce the inflammatory impact but can also elevate the nutritional content of your meal.

Rethinking the ingredients and methods used in your favorite recipes allows you to create dishes that support your health and satisfy your palate. This approach will enable you to enjoy the foods you love, knowing that they are nourishing your body and helping you manage inflammation. Through creative modifications and a focus on high-quality, healthful ingredients, your diet can become a primary tool in your fight against inflammation, all while delighting you with flavors you cherish.

Addressing Common Dietary Concerns and Missteps

When you decide to follow an anti-inflammatory diet, it's like setting a course on a serene river; the journey may seem straightforward, but hidden undercurrents and obstacles can sometimes lead you astray, especially when you have a food intolerance or allergy. For example, if you have gluten intolerance, one of the most common pitfalls you could encounter is the over-reliance on processed gluten-free products. While these products are marketed as healthier alternatives, many are packed with refined starches and sugars that can trigger inflammatory responses like traditional gluten-containing products. Instead of purchasing processed gluten-free bread or snacks, focus on naturally gluten-free whole foods like quinoa, sweet potatoes, and fresh vegetables. These provide not only the safety from gluten for those who are intolerant but also the rich nutrients needed to combat inflammation.

Strategic meal planning ensures you get all the necessary nutrients while following an anti-inflammatory diet. When food allergies or food intolerance causes dairy and other food groups, like fish to be limited, it's possible to miss out on essential nutrients like omega-3 fatty acids, fiber, minerals, and vitamins, including calcium and vitamin D. To avoid these gaps, diversify your diet. Add flaxseeds or chia seeds to your meals for a healthy boost of omega-3s. These seeds blend seamlessly into smoothies and yogurts, making them a convenient and nutritious addition to your diet. For calcium and vitamin D, turn to fortified plant-based milks and mushrooms grown under UV light. If you're concerned about your nutrient levels, consider consulting a nutritionist who can recommend appropriate supplements or dietary adjustments to ensure your nutritional needs are fully met without compromising the anti-inflammatory integrity of your diet.

Mistakes happen, and in the world of dietary management, an accidental slip-up in which you consume inflammatory foods is almost inevitable. Whether it's a bite of a dessert at a party or a sauce you didn't realize contained inflammatory ingredients, it's important not to let this derail your efforts. Instead, focus on minimizing the impact of this mishap. Hydrate well to help your body process and quickly eliminate any inflammatory agents. Engaging in mild physical activity, such as walking, can help boost your metabolism and manage blood sugar spikes. Then, resume your anti-inflammatory eating plan without any guilt. Remember, a single misstep isn't a measure of your overall success; it's the sum of your ongoing efforts that truly counts.

Lastly, embracing continuous learning and adaptation in your dietary habits is vital. The field of nutritional science is constantly evolving, with new studies and data emerging that could influence the effectiveness of an anti-inflammatory diet. Stay informed by regularly reviewing the latest research and dietary recommendations. Subscribe to health and nutrition newsletters, follow relevant medical and health experts on social media, or join health-focused groups where such information is shared and discussed. This habit of continuous learning will deepen your understanding and empower you to make informed decisions about your diet and health, ensuring that your anti-inflammatory diet evolves in alignment with the most current scientific guidance.

Navigating an anti-inflammatory diet requires more than knowing what to eat and what to avoid. It involves understanding the broader nutritional landscape, including how to compensate for potential nutrient deficiencies and handle the inevitable dietary slip-ups. By equipping yourself with this knowledge and remaining adaptable to new information, you can ensure that your diet remains effective, enjoyable, and aligned with your health goals.

Reassessing and Adjusting Your Diet over Time

Adapting to an anti-inflammatory diet is akin to nurturing a garden; it requires attention, care, and occasional adjustments based on how things grow and respond to the environment. Similarly, as you nurture your body with anti-inflammatory foods, staying attuned to how your body reacts and making the necessary adjustments is vital. This ongoing process ensures that your dietary habits consistently align with your health needs and lifestyle changes.

Monitoring Body Responses

To effectively tailor your diet, begin by observing how your body responds to different foods. Note any changes in your symptoms or general well-being after eating certain foods. For instance, you may find that certain oils or nuts trigger discomfort or digestive issues despite being healthy. Keeping a food diary can provide incredible insights here. Record what you eat, the quantities, and how you feel afterward. Identify trends to discern which foods are your partners in reducing inflammation and which counteract your efforts. This vigilant monitoring can serve as a powerful tool, guiding you to refine your diet more precisely to suit your body's unique needs.

It's also helpful to pay attention to broader indicators of health, such as energy levels, sleep quality, skin condition, and digestion. Improvements in these areas can often be a sign that your anti-inflammatory diet is working well. Conversely, if issues in these areas persist or worsen, it might be a cue to reevaluate your dietary choices. Remember, the goal is to reduce inflammation and enhance overall health and vitality.

When to Revise Your Plan

Knowing when to adjust your dietary plan is essential for maintaining its effectiveness. Significant life changes, such as age, stress levels, activity changes, or even climate, can affect your body's nutritional needs. For example, ramping up your exercise routine may call for a boost in protein and carbohydrates to fuel energy and facilitate recovery. Conversely, as you age, it may be helpful to fine-tune your calorie consumption and ensure your diet is rich in nutrients to meet your body's changing needs.

Additionally, keep abreast of new scientific findings that might influence dietary advice. Nutrition science continually evolves, and staying informed can help you make the most beneficial choices. For example, a new study might reveal more in-depth insights into how certain spices can curb inflammation or how gut microbiota interacts with different foods to influence health. These insights should prompt a reassessment of your eating habits, ensuring they remain aligned with the latest research and your health objectives.

Seeking Professional Help

While adjusting your diet on your own is feasible, certain situations call for professional guidance. If your inflammatory symptoms continue or escalate despite following an anti-inflammatory diet, or if you're dealing with the complexities of conditions like autoimmune disorders or major food allergies, consulting a healthcare provider or a registered dietitian is essential. Their expertise is crucial for personalized advice and adjustments to your dietary plan, ensuring it effectively addresses your specific health needs and challenges. Their specialized guidance and personalized support are invaluable in refining your dietary strategy to address your unique health needs and challenges better.

Professionals can help pinpoint specific dietary triggers that you might have overlooked, suggest tests to uncover underlying issues, or develop a personalized eating plan that considers your medical history and nutritional needs. This step is particularly important if you find yourself struggling to balance your nutrient intake or if you need to significantly alter your diet to address health changes.

Long-Term Mindset

Viewing an anti-inflammatory diet as a long-term lifestyle commitment rather than a temporary intervention is essential for sustained success. This perspective encourages ongoing, gradual improvements rather than drastic, short-term changes that are difficult to maintain. Incorporate flexibility within your dietary framework, allowing yourself to adapt to life's changes and enjoy occasional indulgences without guilt. This flexible approach helps integrate the anti-inflammatory diet into your lifestyle more seamlessly, making it a sustainable part of your journey toward optimal health.

Continually monitoring your body's responses, knowing when to revise your plan, seeking professional advice when needed, and maintaining a long-term mindset ensure that your anti-inflammatory diet remains effective and responsive to your evolving health needs. This proactive and adaptive approach helps manage inflammation and supports a balanced, healthy life.

As you move forward, remember that each step you take is not just about avoiding certain foods but about creating a vibrant spectrum of health and vitality that colors every aspect of your life. In the next chapter, we'll explore the broader lifestyle habits that complement your dietary efforts in managing inflammation and improving your well-being.

Make a Difference with Your Review
Unlock the Power of Generosity

"Money can't buy happiness, but giving it away can."

— Freddie Mercury

People who give without expectation live longer, happier lives and make more money. So, if we've got a shot at that during our time together, darn it, I'm going to try.

To make that happen, I have a question for you...

Would you help someone you've never met, even if you never got credit for it?

Who is this person, you ask? They are like you. Or, at least, like you used to be. Less experienced with anti-inflammatory strategies, wanting to make a difference, and needing help, but are not sure where to look.

My mission is to make *The Practical Anti-Inflammatory Diet Guide for Beginners* accessible to everyone. Everything I do stems from that mission. And the only way for me to accomplish that mission is by reaching…well...everyone.

This is where you come in. Most people do, in fact, judge a book by its cover (and its reviews). So, here's my ask on behalf of a struggling chronic inflammation sufferer you've never met:

Please help that chronic inflammation sufferer by leaving a review for this book.

Your gift costs no money and less than 60 seconds to make real but can change a fellow chronic inflammation sufferer's life forever. Your review could help…...one more small business provide for their community. ...one more entrepreneur support their family. ...one more employee get meaningful work. ...one more client transform their life. ...one more dream come true.

To get that 'feel good' feeling and help this person for real, all you have to do is...and it takes less than 60 seconds...leave a review.

Simply scan the QR code below to leave your review:

If you feel good about helping a faceless chronic inflammation sufferer, you are my kind of person. Welcome to the club. You're one of us.

I'm that much more excited to help you manage inflammation and help you enhance your overall well-being more easily than you can possibly imagine. You'll love the strategies I'm about to share in the coming chapters.

Thank you from the bottom of my heart. Now, back to our regularly scheduled programming.

- Your biggest fan, Caroline Green Chow

P.S. Fun fact: If you provide something of value to another person, it makes you more valuable to them. If you'd like goodwill straight from another chronic inflammation sufferer - and you believe this book will help them - send this book their way.

Beyond Diet: Lifestyle Changes for Managing Inflammation

While embracing an anti-inflammatory diet is a decisive step toward managing chronic inflammation, it's only one piece of the puzzle. Integrating regular physical activity into your lifestyle can significantly amplify the benefits of your dietary choices. This chapter delves into how different forms of exercise can help control inflammation. It offers tailored strategies to incorporate more movement into your everyday life to ensure these activities enhance your health without overwhelming your schedule.

The Importance of Regular Physical Activity

Regular physical activity is not just a beneficial addition to your routine; it's a cornerstone of good health and a powerful tool for reducing inflammation. Scientific studies consistently show that exercise helps lower the production of inflammatory markers, such as C-reactive protein (CRP) and interleukin-6 (IL-6) while boosting the release of anti-inflammatory substances in the body. For instance, a study published in the *Journal of Inflammation Research* highlighted a significant reduction in CRP levels among individuals who participated in moderate aerobic exercise over a six-month period. The biological mechanisms behind this involve reducing adipose tissue (which produces inflammatory cytokines) and enhancing the body's antioxidant defenses, which play a critical role in neutralizing free radicals that can trigger inflammation.

When considering the types of exercise most beneficial for managing inflammation, a balanced approach that includes aerobic activities, strength training, and flexibility exercises is ideal. Aerobic exercise, such as brisk walking, cycling, or swimming, helps improve cardiovascular health and aids in weight management, both crucial for reducing inflammation. On the other hand, strength training is effective for building muscle mass, helps regulate blood sugar levels, and improves metabolic health, further aiding in inflammation control. Flexibility exercises, including yoga and stretching routines, contribute by enhancing joint mobility and reducing muscular stiffness, which can be particularly beneficial for those with inflammatory conditions like arthritis.

It's important to remember that not everyone can jump into a high-intensity workout regime, especially if dealing with chronic pain or mobility issues. Customize your exercise routine to fit your individual health conditions and fitness level. Begin by assessing your current fitness level—perhaps consulting a healthcare provider or a fitness professional—and gradually incorporate activities that you enjoy and can perform consistently without discomfort. For instance, if you are new to exercise or have joint issues, starting with low-impact activities like swimming or yoga can be a great way to exercise without putting undue stress on your body.

Including more physical activity in your daily life is simpler than you might think. It doesn't necessarily mean carving out large blocks of time for the gym or long workout sessions. It can be as simple as making small, manageable changes in your routine. Consider walking or cycling to work or opt for the stairs instead of the elevator. If you spend a lot of time at a desk, taking short, frequent breaks to stand or walk around can also help. Active hobbies, such as gardening or dancing, provide another enjoyable way to increase physical activity while enriching your life. These simple changes can make a huge difference in your physical activity levels and help you manage inflammation more effectively.

By understanding the link between exercise and inflammation and tailoring your activities to your unique needs, you can significantly enhance your body's ability to manage inflammation. Regular physical activity supports the efforts of your anti-inflammatory diet and also contributes to overall better health. Regular exercise gives you the strength and vitality to enjoy a full, active life. As you incorporate these practices into your daily routine, remember that consistency is key. Each step you take, no matter how small, is a positive move toward better health and well-being, reducing inflammation and improving your quality of life one activity at a time.

Stress Reduction Techniques That Work

The relationship between stress and inflammation is more significant than many people might assume. When you experience stress, your body responds by releasing hormones like cortisol and adrenaline, which are part of your fight-or-flight response. While these hormones are crucial in acute situations, their presence for extended periods due to chronic stress can lead to increased inflammation. Chronic stress disrupts many of your body's natural functions, increasing susceptibility to inflammation and related conditions.

Therefore, managing stress is critical for maintaining mental wellness and as a primary strategy in mitigating chronic inflammation.

Incorporating mindfulness meditation, yoga, and deep breathing exercises into your daily routine can be extremely beneficial to manage stress effectively. Mindfulness meditation involves sitting quietly and paying attention to thoughts, sounds, breathing sensations, or body parts, bringing your attention to the present without drifting into concerns about the past or future. This practice can help reduce the stress hormone cortisol, thereby lowering inflammation. Research has shown that regular mindfulness meditation can significantly reduce the body's inflammatory markers, making it a powerful tool in your stress management arsenal.

Yoga, which combines physical postures, breath control, and meditation, can also relieve stress effectively. By improving your body's flexibility and balance, yoga can help release the physical tension that accumulates during periods of stress. The breathing techniques practiced in yoga can enhance your lung capacity and trigger your body's relaxation response, reducing stress and potentially lowering inflammation. Yoga's meditative components also contribute to improved mental focus and calmness, further aiding in stress reduction.

Deep breathing exercises are another simple yet powerful method to manage stress. By focusing on slow, deep, and consistent breaths, you can stimulate your body's parasympathetic nervous system, which opposes the stress-induced responses of the sympathetic nervous system. Deep breathing not only relaxes the body by reducing heart rate and blood pressure but also helps detoxify the body and reduce acidity, which is linked to inflammation.

Developing a routine integrating these stress reduction techniques can make managing stress more accessible and practical. Start by setting aside a specific time each day for these practices, even if it's just for five to ten minutes. Gradually, as these activities become a habit, you may find it easier to extend the duration or add additional sessions throughout your day. For instance, beginning your day with yoga can energize and prepare you for the day ahead, while ending your day with mindfulness meditation might help you unwind and improve sleep quality.

Assessing the effectiveness of these stress reduction techniques is important to ensure they meet your personal needs. Keep a journal to record your stress levels and any symptoms of inflammation you experience daily. Note any changes as you incorporate these practices into your life. Over time, look for patterns that indicate improvement, such as reduced pain or increased feelings of well-being. If a particular practice does not help after a few weeks, consider trying a different method or adjusting the frequency and duration of your current practice. Remember, the goal is to find what works best for you and your lifestyle, allowing you to manage stress effectively and reduce its impact on your overall health and well-being.

Understanding the profound impact of stress on inflammation and embracing effective techniques to manage stress equip you with crucial tools to enhance both your mental and physical health. These practices are vital in managing existing inflammatory conditions and preventing potential health issues related to chronic stress and inflammation. As you continue to explore these techniques, remember that consistency is vital—regular practice can yield significant benefits, helping you lead a healthier and more balanced life.

The Impact of Sleep on Inflammation

A good night's sleep is often touted as the best medicine, but it's not just an old wives' tale—there's robust science behind the effects of sleep on your physical health, particularly regarding inflammation. When you sleep, your body goes through processes of repair and rejuvenation, which include regulating the levels of various inflammatory mediators in your bloodstream. Insufficient or poor-quality sleep can disrupt these processes, leading to increased inflammatory responses. This exacerbation is often seen in the form of elevated cytokine levels and increased stress hormones, which can persist throughout the day, potentially leading to chronic inflammation and associated disorders such as cardiovascular diseases and diabetes.

You can implement several actionable strategies to create a restful environment in order to improve your sleep quality and duration. First, consider the physical setup of your bedroom. It should be a sanctuary to promote sleep, which means comfortable bedding, minimal noise, and optimal temperature settings. Using heavy curtains or an eye mask can block out light, while earplugs can help manage unwanted noise. Additionally, the temperature of your room can significantly affect sleep quality. Most people sleep best in a relatively cool room, around 65 degrees Fahrenheit (18 degrees Celsius), with adequate ventilation.

Establishing regular sleep-wake cycles is also crucial. Target going to bed and waking up at the same time every day, even on weekends. This consistency helps regulate your body's internal clock and can help you fall asleep and wake up more naturally. You must avoid stimulants like caffeine and nicotine close to bedtime, as they can disrupt sleep. Similarly, while alcohol may help you relax, it can interfere with your sleep cycle once you're asleep. Also, consider limiting naps, especially in the late afternoon or evening, as they can hinder nighttime sleep.

Common sleep disorders like sleep apnea and insomnia can significantly impact your inflammation levels. Sleep apnea, where breathing stops and starts repeatedly, can lead to fragmented sleep and low oxygen levels in the blood, causing or exacerbating systemic inflammation. Insomnia, which can involve difficulty falling or staying asleep, may lead to chronic sleep deprivation, another pathway to increased inflammation. If you suspect you have a sleep disorder, it's critical that you seek professional help. Treatments are available, and they can markedly improve your sleep quality and potentially reduce inflammation. For sleep apnea, options include CPAP machines or lifestyle changes, while insomnia may be managed with cognitive-behavioral therapy for insomnia (CBT-I) or, in some cases, medication.

Monitoring your sleep patterns can also play a pivotal role in managing inflammation. Numerous tools and apps are available that you can use to track the duration and quality of your sleep, providing insights into patterns or habits that could be having a negative impact on your sleep. These tools often monitor sleep stages, interruptions, and overall sleep quality, offering detailed feedback that can help you make informed adjustments to your sleep habits. For instance, you might discover that consuming heavy meals or exercising late in the day disrupts your sleep, and adjusting these behaviors could lead to improvements in both sleep and inflammation markers.

Understanding the intricate relationship between sleep and inflammation and taking proactive steps to enhance sleep quality will equip you with another vital tool for managing inflammation. Adequate, restful sleep helps modulate inflammatory responses and supports overall health, improving everything from mood and energy levels to cognitive function. As you refine your sleep habits and create an environment conducive to restorative sleep, you'll probably notice improvements in your alertness and mood and the systemic health markers that contribute to a vibrant, active life.

Hydration: Your Secret Weapon Against Inflammation

Proper hydration plays a pivotal role in maintaining optimal health, especially when controlling inflammation. Every cell in your body relies on water to function efficiently. Without adequate hydration, your body cannot effectively flush out toxins and waste products, which can contribute to inflammation. When cells are dehydrated, they don't function as well, and this can lead to an increase in the production of cytokines and inflammatory markers that can make conditions like arthritis and other inflammatory diseases worse. Additionally, sufficient hydration helps to maintain the health of your lymphatic system, a critical component of your immune system that helps to clear away waste and toxins from your body. By keeping this system running smoothly, you can help prevent the buildup of inflammatory substances in your body.

The amount of water people need can vary greatly and depends on individual factors such as weight, activity level, and the climate you live in. A general guideline is to aim for about half an ounce to an ounce of water per pound of body weight each day. For example, if you weigh 130 pounds, that would be 65 to 130 ounces of water daily. However, it's important to adjust this amount based on your activity level and environmental conditions. If you're physically active or if you live in a hot climate, you may need to increase water intake to compensate for the incremental fluid loss through sweat. Conversely, your intake might be on the lower end of the range in cooler climates or during less active periods.

Incorporating hydrating foods into your diet is another effective strategy to maintain optimal hydration levels. Foods like cucumbers, melons, and leafy greens are high in water content and provide a rich source of anti-inflammatory nutrients such as vitamins, minerals, and antioxidants. Cucumbers, for instance, are about 95 percent water and can be a refreshing addition to salads or a hydrating snack. Melons, including watermelon, cantaloupe, and honeydew, are also excellent for boosting hydration due to their high water content and beneficial nutrients like vitamin C and potassium, which support immune function and reduce inflammation. Leafy greens like spinach, kale, and lettuce contribute not only to hydration but also to essential nutrients like iron, calcium, and phytonutrients that contain anti-inflammatory properties.

Avoiding dehydration is crucial, especially during physical activity or hot weather, when your body loses fluids more rapidly. Recognizing the signs of dehydration can help you take proactive steps to maintain hydration. Common symptoms include thirst, dry mouth, fatigue, light-headedness, and darker-colored urine. If you experience these symptoms, that's a signal from your body that you need to increase your fluid intake. Drinking fluids regularly throughout the day is advisable to prevent dehydration, not just when you feel thirsty. Carrying a water bottle with you as a reminder to drink periodically can be helpful. Additionally, starting your day with a glass of water and drinking a glass before each meal can ensure you're well-hydrated throughout the day.

By understanding hydration's crucial role in controlling inflammation and implementing strategies to ensure you're adequately hydrated, you support your body's natural ability to fight inflammation. This strategy helps manage existing inflammation and boosts your overall health and energy, ensuring your body functions at its best and leaving you feeling refreshed and rejuvenated. Remember, staying hydrated isn't just about drinking plenty of water; it also means incorporating foods high in water content into your diet and being mindful of your body's signals.

Supplements and Natural Remedies

Although diet and lifestyle adjustments play a critical role in managing chronic inflammation, they sometimes need a little boost. Under these circumstances, supplements and natural remedies can play a supportive part. Integrating certain supplements known for their anti-inflammatory properties can provide additional benefits that help manage inflammation more effectively.

- Omega-3 fatty acids found abundantly in fish oil have been widely researched and shown to reduce the production of substances linked to inflammation. Studies have highlighted that omega-3s can significantly decrease the production of specific inflammatory markers, such as cytokines and eicosanoids.
- Turmeric, which contains the active compound curcumin, has strong anti-inflammatory properties that have been celebrated in both traditional and modern medicine. Curcumin helps to inhibit molecules that play a role in inflammation. Its efficacy can be comparable to some anti-inflammatory medications, generally without the side effects.
- Another potent natural anti-inflammatory is ginger, which contains gingerol, a potent anti-inflammatory and antioxidant. Ginger is known to reduce inflammation

associated with conditions like osteoarthritis and rheumatism. It works by inhibiting the synthesis of pro-inflammatory cytokines and chemokines, providing relief from inflammation-driven pain and swelling.

While the benefits are significant, it's essential to approach supplementation with care. Always choose high-quality supplements and adhere to the recommended dosages to maximize benefits and minimize potential side effects. For instance, with fish oil, a general recommendation is to aim for about one to three grams daily. Of course, this can vary based on individual health conditions and needs.

When considering supplements, it's important to consult a healthcare provider before starting any new regimen, especially if you have underlying health conditions or are taking other medications. Consultation ensures that any supplements you take do not interfere with other treatments and are designed to effectively support your specific health requirements.

Natural topical remedies can be highly effective for localized inflammation, such as skin irritations or joint pain. Aloe vera, for example, is well known for its soothing and anti-inflammatory properties. Applying aloe vera gel to inflamed skin can help reduce redness and swelling, promoting healing. CBD oil is another topical treatment that has gained popularity for its anti-inflammatory and pain-relief properties. When applied to the skin, it interacts with the cannabinoid receptors in the immune cells, reducing inflammation and providing relief.

Herbal teas can also support inflammation management when included in your daily routine. Teas like green tea contain high levels of catechins, antioxidants that reduce inflammatory responses. Drinking a few cups of green tea each day can help lower inflammation and bestow other health benefits, such as improved heart health and enhanced metabolic rates. Chamomile tea is another excellent choice for its calming and anti-inflammatory effects, making it a perfect beverage to unwind in the evening. It reduces stress and inflammation simultaneously. Willow bark tea is often called nature's aspirin, except it is gentler on the stomach. It contains salicin, which is converted by the body to salicylic acid, providing relief from pain and inflammation.

When used correctly and with a balanced anti-inflammatory diet and lifestyle, these natural remedies and supplements can greatly enhance your ability to manage inflammation. They provide natural, often safer alternatives to pharmaceutical interventions and empower you to take control of your health holistically. As you explore these options, remember that consistency and quality are key—regular use of these remedies as part of an overall health plan can yield the best results, helping you lead a healthier and more vibrant life free from the constraints of chronic inflammation.

Building a Support System for Long-Term Success

Embarking on the journey toward an anti-inflammatory lifestyle brings immense rewards but can also seem daunting when tackled solo. A supportive community is important. More than just being beneficial, a robust support network is essential for successfully adopting and maintaining lifestyle changes that yield long-term health improvements. Social support provides emotional encouragement and helps people stick to their dietary goals. It also directly contributes to better physical health by reducing stress, a key driver of inflammation.

The impact of social support extends across various aspects of health management. Studies have shown that individuals who feel a greater sense of community and support are more likely to stick to their health goals. They experience less stress and better overall health outcomes. It is particularly true when making significant lifestyle changes, such as altering long-held eating habits or incorporating new physical activities. These can be challenging to sustain over time without encouragement and accountability. Engaging with supportive friends, family, or community members can make these transitions more enjoyable and less overwhelming, fostering a positive environment that encourages persistence.

Finding the right community resources can be pivotal. Many communities offer support groups, fitness classes, or clubs focused on healthy living, which can be invaluable resources. These groups provide a platform to meet others who share similar goals and challenges, offering an opportunity to exchange tips, share recipes, and provide mutual encouragement. Additionally, many support groups are led by professionals who can provide expert guidance and help navigate the complexities of managing chronic inflammation. To locate these resources, consider checking with local health clinics, community centers, or online platforms dedicated to health and wellness.

It's important to involve your family and friends in your journey toward an anti-inflammatory lifestyle. Sharing your goals with loved ones not only helps them understand your aspirations but also opens up avenues for their support. This collaborative effort could lead to the introduction of anti-inflammatory meals that everyone enjoys or the organization of group activities like cycling or hiking. Such engagement strengthens your commitment to your health goals and encourages those around you to adopt healthier habits, creating a ripple effect of wellness in your community.

Additionally, building a network of healthcare professionals who are knowledgeable about anti-inflammatory lifestyles can provide a foundation of expert support. This network may include nutritionists who can customize your diet to meet your specific needs, personal trainers who can design unique exercise programs that don't exacerbate your condition, and therapists who can help address the psychological aspects of long-term health management. These professionals can offer the specialized guidance needed to navigate the complexities of reducing inflammation through lifestyle changes, providing informed and tailored support to your individual set of circumstances.

By cultivating a supportive network, you're not just gaining allies in your journey to reduce inflammation—you're enhancing your capacity to sustain positive changes over the long haul. This support network can become a powerful motivational force, helping you overcome obstacles and celebrating your successes along the way. As you continue to develop and nurture these relationships, you'll find that managing your inflammation becomes a more integrated and enjoyable part of your life, filled with shared experiences and collective victories.

As we conclude this chapter, remember that the journey of managing inflammation is not just about the foods you eat or the exercises you perform; it's also about the people you surround yourself with. These relationships can empower you to maintain your commitments, inspire you to overcome challenges and provide a source of comfort and motivation throughout your health journey. In the next chapter, we'll explore advanced topics in anti-inflammatory living, diving deeper into specific conditions and innovative management strategies that can further enhance your quality of life, ensuring that every step you take is supported by sound science and a community that cares.

Advanced Topics in Anti-Inflammatory Living

The Truth about Nightshades and Inflammation

As you delve deeper into the intricacies of an anti-inflammatory lifestyle, it's important to explore some of the more nuanced aspects of diet that might be influencing your inflammation levels. One such topic that often stirs debate is the role of nightshades in the diet. Nightshades are a diverse group of plants that include common vegetables like tomatoes, peppers, eggplants, and potatoes. These staples of many diets are grouped together because they belong to the Solanaceae family, which shares specific biological characteristics and chemical compounds.

Identifying Nightshades

Nightshades can be found in many kitchens and are beloved for their versatility in cooking. Tomatoes, for instance, are essential for their juicy acidity in salads and sauces; peppers brighten dishes with their crisp texture and vibrant colors; eggplants offer a meaty texture perfect for hearty meals; and potatoes are a global staple, beloved in a myriad of culinary traditions. Despite their popularity, these vegetables share a common feature that might impact individuals with sensitivity to certain chemical compounds they contain.

Why Nightshades Might Cause Inflammation

The primary concern with nightshades is related to their content of elements such as solanine, a glycoalkaloid that can elicit an inflammatory response in some people. Solanine is part of the plant's natural defenses, serving as a deterrent to pests and diseases. In sensitive individuals, these compounds can interfere with enzymes in the muscles, potentially leading to discomfort and inflammation. Additionally, nightshades contain lectins, proteins that can bind to cell membranes and have been suggested to increase intestinal permeability, potentially leading to an inflammatory response known as "leaky gut."

Research Findings

The scientific community remains divided on the definitive impact of nightshades on inflammation. Some studies suggest that, in individuals with specific health conditions such as rheumatoid arthritis or other autoimmune diseases, eliminating nightshades can lead to noticeable improvements in symptoms. For example, a survey conducted by the Arthritis Foundation found that some people reported a reduction in joint pain when avoiding nightshades. However, comprehensive clinical studies are limited, and more research is needed to fully understand the connection between nightshades and inflammation.

Personal Tolerance Assessment

Given the mixed evidence, the best approach if you suspect that nightshades might be affecting your inflammation is to conduct a personal assessment through an elimination diet. Remove nightshades from your diet for a period—usually around three to four weeks—while monitoring any changes in symptoms. After this period, reintroduce them one at a time, noting any changes in symptoms. This method can help you determine whether nightshades trigger an inflammatory response and whether you should limit or avoid them in your diet.

Navigating the complexities of which foods support your health and which might hinder it can be challenging. However, the potential benefits of an anti-inflammatory diet, such as reduced discomfort and improved well-being, can be a source of hope and motivation. By understanding and listening to your body's signals, you can tailor your dietary choices to support a life free from inflammation-driven discomfort. Remember, the goal of an anti-inflammatory diet is not just to eliminate certain foods but to find a balance that works uniquely for your body, enhancing your health and well-being.

Alcohol and Inflammation: What You Need to Know

When contemplating the effects of diet on inflammation, alcohol is a topic that cannot be overlooked. Its consumption can have complex impacts on your body, influencing everything from your digestive system to your immune response. Understanding these effects is crucial if you aim to manage inflammation effectively. By being informed and aware, you can make conscious choices about your consumption and its potential impact on your health. Excessive alcohol intake is linked to adverse health outcomes, particularly concerning inflammation.

Alcohol can affect bodily systems in numerous ways, and one of its most significant impacts is on the liver, which is crucial to managing inflammation. The liver helps to filter toxins from your body and aids in the regulation of inflammation. When you consume alcohol, your liver gives priority to metabolizing the alcohol over other tasks. Consequently, fatty acids can accumulate in the liver cells, causing a condition known as alcoholic fatty liver. This condition can progress to more severe liver inflammation, known as alcoholic hepatitis, and eventually to irreversible damage or cirrhosis. Alcohol can disrupt the balance of your gut microbiome, increasing intestinal permeability and allowing more endotoxins to enter the bloodstream, which can induce systemic inflammation.

The concept of moderation is particularly pertinent when discussing alcohol consumption in the context of inflammation. Typically, moderate drinking is defined as up to one drink per day for women and up to two drinks per day for men. Exceeding these moderate amounts can lead to an increased risk of chronic inflammation and related diseases like heart disease, diabetes, and various cancers.

A deeper dive into the types of alcohol makes it clear that their impact on inflammation can be very unfavorable. Liquors and beers, which are high in sugars and certain additives, may contribute significantly to inflammatory processes. Beer, for instance, contains gluten, which creates a problem for individuals with gluten sensitivities or celiac disease, potentially triggering inflammatory responses.

Adhering to guidelines for moderate consumption is pivotal for those who choose to include alcohol in their diet. Opting for drinks lower in sugar and additives can also minimize their impact on inflammation. When consuming alcohol, it's beneficial to pair it with foods that can mitigate its effects, such as those rich in fiber and protein. Additionally, ensuring adequate hydration by drinking water alongside alcoholic beverages can help counteract the diuretic effect of alcohol, supporting overall hydration status and reducing potential inflammatory responses.

In essence, while moderate alcohol consumption can fit into an anti-inflammatory lifestyle, it requires careful consideration. By understanding how different alcoholic beverages affect your body and making informed choices, you can enjoy these drinks in a way that aligns with your health goals, particularly in managing inflammation effectively.

Dairy: Friend or Foe in an Anti-Inflammatory Diet?

Understanding the impact of dairy on an anti-inflammatory diet can be complex, given its widespread consumption and nutritional value, including essential calcium and protein. Yet, dairy's effect on inflammation is not one-size-fits-all, mainly due to individual variations in digestion and tolerance, such as lactose intolerance and milk allergies.

Lactose Intolerance versus Milk Allergy

Understanding the distinction between lactose intolerance and milk allergy is crucial for identifying their impacts on inflammation. The sugar in milk and dairy products is called lactose. Lactose intolerance involves difficulty digesting lactose due to a deficiency in lactase, the enzyme responsible for breaking down this sugar in the digestive system. Lactose intolerance can produce symptoms such as bloating, diarrhea, and gas, but it does not typically trigger an inflammatory response unless it results in significant digestive distress. On the other hand, a milk allergy involves an immune system reaction to one or more of the proteins present in milk, such as casein or whey. This reaction can cause inflammation as the body perceives these proteins as harmful invaders, leading to a wide range of symptoms, from hives and itching to severe anaphylaxis.

Pro-Inflammatory versus Anti-Inflammatory Properties of Dairy

The debate over dairy's role in inflammation is ongoing, with studies yielding mixed results. Some research suggests that specific components of dairy, particularly the saturated fats found in whole milk and cheese, may contribute to inflammation, particularly in individuals already susceptible to inflammatory diseases. Conversely, other studies indicate that fermented dairy products like yogurt and kefir may have anti-inflammatory effects due to their probiotic content, which supports gut health and reduces inflammation. Moreover, dairy products are sources of crucial nutrients like vitamin D and calcium, both of which are instrumental in regulating the body's inflammatory processes.

Given this complex landscape, it's not surprising that dairy's impact on inflammation can be both individual and context-dependent. For some, especially those with a diagnosed dairy allergy or significant lactose intolerance, avoiding dairy may be beneficial in managing inflammation; for those who can tolerate dairy without digestive issues, including specific dairy products in their diet may contribute to anti-inflammatory advantages.

Alternative Dairy Options

For those looking to reduce or avoid dairy due to personal health responses or preferences, numerous non-dairy alternatives can serve as part of an anti-inflammatory diet. Almond, soy, coconut, and oat milk are popular plant-based options. Each of these alternatives comes with its own set of nutritional profiles and potential health benefits. For instance, almond milk is typically lower in calories and fat than cow's milk but high in vitamin E, an antioxidant that can help combat inflammation. Coconut milk is rich in medium-chain triglycerides (MCTs), fats the body can easily convert into energy and may help reduce inflammation. Soy milk offers a protein content comparable to cow's milk and contains isoflavones, compounds known for their anti-inflammatory properties.

When choosing non-dairy alternatives, it's essential to opt for unsweetened varieties to avoid the added sugars that can exacerbate inflammation. Additionally, checking labels for fortification can help ensure you get all the essential nutrients like calcium and vitamins D and B12, which are naturally present in cow's milk and are necessary for overall health.

Personalized Dairy Consumption Plan

Deciding whether to include dairy in your diet should be based on your individual health responses and nutritional needs. If you suspect that dairy is impacting your inflammation or overall health, consider conducting an elimination diet by removing dairy from your diet for a few weeks and monitoring any changes in symptoms. Reintroduce dairy gradually, noting any reactions as you add different types of dairy back into your diet. This approach can help you determine your tolerance levels and whether certain forms of dairy are more problematic than others.

Incorporating moderate amounts of dairy can contribute to a balanced diet for those who tolerate dairy well and exhibit no adverse inflammatory responses. Choosing low-fat or fermented dairy products can maximize the nutritional benefits while minimizing potential inflammatory effects. Maintaining a varied diet with large quantities of fruits, vegetables, whole grains, and lean proteins alongside dairy can help ensure a comprehensive intake of anti-inflammatory nutrients.

In conclusion, the role of dairy in an anti-inflammatory diet is nuanced and highly personal. By understanding your body's responses and making informed choices about the types of dairy or alternatives you consume, you can effectively manage inflammation and support your overall health. Whether you choose to include dairy or opt for non-dairy options, the key is to prioritize natural, nutrient-rich foods that foster a balanced and health-supportive diet.

The Role of Fats: Omega-3s versus Omega-6s

In the context of an anti-inflammatory diet, understanding the different types of dietary fats—particularly omega-3 and omega-6 fatty acids—is crucial. These fats are not just energy sources; they play significant roles in your body's inflammatory processes. Omega-3 fatty acids are known to be anti-inflammatory. They help reduce the production of inflammation-related substances, such as eicosanoids and cytokines. Conversely, despite being essential, omega-6 fatty acids can encourage inflammation when their intake disproportionately exceeds that of omega-3s.

Omega-3 fatty acids are primarily found in fish, such as salmon, mackerel, and sardines, which are rich in EPA (eicosapentaenoic acid) and DHA (docosahexaenoic acid), two potent forms of omega-3s. These substances are crucial for brain function, growth, and development. Plant-based sources include flaxseeds, chia seeds, and walnuts. They contain ALA (alpha-linolenic acid), another type of omega-3 fatty acid that the body partially converts to EPA and DHA. Omega-6 fatty acids, on the other hand, are prevalent in many vegetable oils like corn oil, safflower oil, sunflower oil, and nuts and seeds.

The modern diet, however, tends to be disproportionately heavy in omega-6 fatty acids relative to omega-3s. This imbalance is a concern because excessive levels of omega-6 fatty acids can lead to the production of pro-inflammatory chemicals. Traditionally, the human diet maintained a more balanced ratio of omega-6 to omega-3 fatty acids, roughly equal in proportion. However, modern dietary patterns have shifted this balance dramatically, with current ratios leaning as much as 16:1 in favor of omega-6s. This significant discrepancy correlates with increased inflammation-related conditions, including heart disease and arthritis.

The consequences of this fatty acid imbalance extend beyond mere numbers. A diet high in omega-6s and low in omega-3s can exacerbate inflammatory processes and may contribute to developing chronic diseases. Inflammatory responses are a natural part of the body's immune system. However, when inflammation goes unchecked due to dietary imbalances, it can lead to chronic inflammation, which is linked to a host of health issues, including cardiovascular diseases, type 2 diabetes, obesity, and autoimmune diseases.

To optimize your fatty acid intake, it is advisable to focus on increasing omega-3s while managing omega-6s. It is vital to achieve a healthier balance between these fatty acids and not eliminate omega-6s, as they are essential for good health. You can increase your dietary intake of omega-3s by including more fatty fish in your meals. Plan to have two to three servings of fatty fish per week. For vegetarians or those who prefer plant-based sources of food, options such as flaxseeds, chia seeds, and walnuts are beneficial. To further balance the scale, consider reducing your use of certain vegetable oils high in omega-6s in cooking and food preparation, switching instead to oils with an improved balance of omega-3 to omega-6 ratio, such as olive oil or flaxseed oil.

Adapting your diet to favor a balance of omega-3 and omega-6 fatty acids can significantly affect your body's inflammatory status and overall health. By making conscious choices about the types of fats you consume, you empower yourself to manage inflammation more effectively, paving the way for a healthier, more vibrant lifestyle. Remember, the goal is to embrace these changes as part of a sustained commitment to your health and not merely to adjust your diet temporarily. This approach helps manage current inflammation and prevent future health issues associated with chronic inflammation. As you modify your eating habits, pay close attention to your body's reactions. Embrace the empowering journey of transformation as you experience the shift toward a healthier you.

Understanding Food Intolerances and Allergies

Navigating the complex world of food intolerances and allergies is important for anyone aiming to manage chronic inflammation through diet. While both conditions can provoke bodily reactions, understanding their distinct characteristics and how they affect your immune system is essential. A food intolerance generally results from difficulty digesting specific foods, leading to uncomfortable symptoms such as bloating, gas, and diarrhea. Food intolerance does not typically involve the immune system. A food allergy, however, is an immune system response in which the body mistakenly identifies a specific protein found in food as harmful, triggering a protective response. This allergic reaction can cause very serious symptoms, including hives, swelling, and, in extreme cases, anaphylaxis, which can be life-threatening.

The distinction is vital because, while both can cause discomfort, allergies can also drive significant inflammatory responses throughout the body, potentially aggravating symptoms of chronic inflammation. Common food allergy and intolerance triggers include dairy products, gluten-containing grains, nuts, and shellfish. These foods contain proteins or carbohydrates that can be difficult to digest or can trigger immune responses in susceptible individuals.

For those suspecting food intolerances or allergies, the path to diagnosis typically involves a combination of dietary strategies and medical tests. You can use an elimination diet approach to identify offending foods. This involves removing foods suspected of causing symptoms for a period, then gradually reintroducing them one at a time and observing the body's reaction. This method can effectively pinpoint specific foods that cause issues, helping to tailor a diet that avoids triggers. For a more precise diagnosis, especially in the case of allergies, medical tests such as skin prick tests or blood tests measuring immune system responses to particular food proteins can confirm suspicions.

Managing food intolerances and allergies involves more than just avoiding certain foods; it's about adjusting your diet to maintain nutritional balance and enjoyment of eating. Substituting problematic foods with alternatives that provide similar nutritional benefits is key. For instance, those intolerant to cow's milk might turn to fortified plant-based alternatives like almond or soy milk, which provide calcium and vitamin D. Similarly, grains like quinoa, buckwheat, and rice are excellent alternatives for those avoiding gluten.

Living with food intolerances and allergies doesn't mean you have to miss out on delicious and nutritious meals. You can design a diet that meets your nutritional needs and delights your palate with careful planning and a bit of creativity. Focusing on whole, unprocessed foods and incorporating various fruits, vegetables, grains, and protein sources can ensure you benefit from a well-rounded diet. Moreover, embracing the art of cooking can transform dietary restrictions into an opportunity to discover new tastes and textures, turning meal preparation into a rewarding experience that supports your health goals.

Remember the importance of vigilance and education as you adapt to a lifestyle free from your specific food triggers. Reading food labels, asking about ingredients in restaurants, and remaining informed about your condition can help you avoid adverse reactions and proactively manage your health. Over time, these practices become second nature, seamlessly integrating into your daily routine. At this stage, you will enjoy your meals with confidence and peace of mind.

The Power of Spices and Herbs in Your Diet

In the quest to tame chronic inflammation, the culinary world offers a treasure trove of ingredients that enhance flavor and provide significant health benefits. Spices and herbs have been revered throughout history for their medicinal properties, and modern science increasingly supports their role in reducing inflammation.

Turmeric, ginger, cinnamon, and basil stand out not only for their distinctive flavors but also for their potent anti-inflammatory properties.

- Turmeric, often called the golden spice, contains curcumin, a compound with powerful anti-inflammatory and antioxidant properties. Research has shown that curcumin can inhibit key molecules contributing to inflammation, such as cytokines and prostaglandins. Curcumin's ability to calm inflammation is similar to some prescribed anti-inflammatory drugs, making turmeric an essential addition to an anti-inflammatory diet.
- Ginger, another spice with a long medicinal history, works similarly. The active components, such as gingerol, block the synthesis of pro-inflammatory compounds and enhance the production of substances that reduce inflammation. This dual action makes ginger an effective remedy for relieving symptoms associated with inflammation, such as pain and swelling.
- While popularly known for its sweet and warm flavor, cinnamon also packs a potent anti-inflammatory punch. Studies have identified several compounds in cinnamon that reduce inflammation. These compounds inhibit the activity of certain proteins and enzymes that play a role in inflammation, making cinnamon beneficial for its taste and health properties.
- Basil, with its sweet and earthy aroma, contains essential oils such as eugenol. This oil has been shown to block enzymes in the body that cause inflammation, similar to how certain pain relievers work.

Including these spices and herbs in your meals can be both delicious and health-promoting. Turmeric can be added to curries, soups, and even smoothies to bring a warm, earthy flavor and a beautiful golden color. Ginger adds a zesty kick to dishes and can be used fresh in stir-fries, infused into teas, or added to marinades. Cinnamon is versatile enough to spice up both sweet and savory dishes, from oatmeal and baked goods to stews and marinades. You can sprinkle basil over salads, blend it into pesto, or add it to pasta sauces to enhance flavor while providing anti-inflammatory benefits.

While the health benefits of these spices and herbs are compelling, potential interactions and side effects, especially when consumed in large quantities or as concentrated extracts, should be considered.

- High doses of turmeric can cause digestive upset in some people and may interact with blood-thinning medications due to its anti-clotting properties.
- Excessive consumption of cinnamon can lead to liver toxicity due to the presence of coumarin, a natural compound found in some types of cinnamon. Always consult with a healthcare provider before starting any new supplement regimen, especially if you have underlying health conditions or are taking other medications.

Integrating a variety of spices and herbs into your diet is a flavorful way to combat inflammation and enhance overall health. By using these ingredients judiciously, you can enjoy the culinary benefits while tapping into their healing properties. As you continue to explore the vast array of spices and herbs available, you'll enrich your palate and experience a healthier, more vibrant life.

Reflective Journaling Prompt

Reflect on how you currently use spices and herbs in your cooking. Are there new ways you could incorporate anti-inflammatory spices like turmeric, ginger, cinnamon, or basil into your meals? Consider setting a goal to try one new spice or herb each week and note any changes in how you feel.

As we wrap up this exploration of spices and herbs, remember that each small step you take in adjusting your diet contributes to a larger picture of health and well-being. These natural ingredients offer a simple yet effective way to enhance your meals and manage inflammation, paving the way for a healthier lifestyle. Ahead, we will continue to explore other essential aspects of an anti-inflammatory lifestyle, ensuring you have the knowledge and tools to support your health journey.

Motivation and Real-Life Success Stories

Imagine stepping into the shoes of a person who once felt bogged down by the weight of chronic inflammation, who struggled with discomfort and fatigue, only to turn their life around through the transformative power of diet. This chapter is dedicated to real-life warriors who have navigated the challenging waters of dietary change and come out stronger and healthier. Their stories are not just narratives but testaments to the power of perseverance and the tangible benefits of an anti-inflammatory lifestyle. Each account sheds light on the personal battles, strategic triumphs, and profound life changes from embracing this healthful path. These are the stories of people like you, who took control of their well-being and discovered a vibrant new way of life.

Inspiring Stories from Those Who've Made the Change

Diverse Success Narratives

Take, for example, the story of Michael, a retired veteran who battled severe arthritis and chronic back pain for years. His journey began on a small, seemingly insignificant morning when he decided to swap his breakfast bacon for a bowl of oatmeal topped with fresh berries. This simple change marked the start of a journey that saw him gradually phasing out processed foods in favor of whole, anti-inflammatory alternatives. Months into his new diet, Michael noticed a significant decrease in his pain levels and an increase in his mobility. Encouraged by these changes, he continued to explore and integrate more anti-inflammatory foods, eventually reporting a 40 percent reduction in his symptoms and a newfound zest for life.

Then, there's the story of Anita, a middle-aged school teacher and mother of two who suffered from persistent digestive issues and skin flare-ups. Frustrated by the lack of progress with traditional medications, she attended a nutrition workshop that introduced her to the anti-inflammatory diet. Skeptical yet desperate for relief, Anita began incorporating foods rich in omega-3s and antioxidants into her family meals. Not only did her symptoms begin to alleviate, but she also saw remarkable improvements in her children's energy levels and overall health. Her kitchen became her new pharmacy, filled with colorful fruits, vegetables, and grains that became the cornerstone of her family's health.

Challenges and Triumphs

Embracing an anti-inflammatory diet is not without its hurdles. Michael, for instance, initially struggled with cravings for his old comfort foods and found it challenging to maintain his new habits while dining out. However, through trial and error, he learned how to make smarter food choices and how to modify his favorite dishes to fit his new lifestyle. Anita initially faced resistance from her family, as her children missed their usual snacks. But by involving them in the cooking process and experimenting with recipes together, she slowly won them over with tasty, healthy alternatives that everyone enjoyed.

Key Lessons Learned

The key takeaway from these stories is the importance of persistence and adaptability. Dietary changes, especially significant ones like adopting an anti-inflammatory diet, require a commitment to learning and flexibility. Both Michael and Anita had to experiment with different foods and recipes to find what worked best for their unique bodies and lifestyles. They learned to listen to their bodies' cues and adjusted their diets accordingly, which was crucial in successfully adopting the anti-inflammatory lifestyle.

The Transformative Power of Education and Support in Health Journeys

These narratives underscore that while the path to reducing inflammation through diet is personal, you do not have to walk it alone. The successes of others provide a roadmap that can inspire and energize new individuals to begin their journeys toward better health. Each story serves as inspiration, demonstrating how, with dedication and well-informed decisions, anyone can harness the restorative power of nutrition to lessen inflammation and enhance their well-being. The sense of community and support is palpable, making you feel connected and less alone on your health journey.

Tips for Staying Motivated on Your Health Journey

Embarking on a path to better health through an anti-inflammatory diet can be exciting and rewarding, yet maintaining motivation over time sometimes presents a challenge. It's like embarking on a long hike; the initial enthusiasm is often plentiful, but keeping the pace requires some strategy and encouragement as the path stretches out. Here, we will delve into practical ways to stay motivated, from setting achievable goals to handling the inevitable plateaus.

Setting and Tracking Goals

Setting realistic goals is the cornerstone of any successful health transformation. Think of your health goals as your GPS coordinates, guiding your daily decisions and actions. Start with clear, achievable objectives, such as incorporating a serving of vegetables into each meal or replacing one processed snack with a healthier option each day. As these become habitual, you can set more ambitious goals like eliminating refined sugar from your diet or cooking all meals at home during weekdays. Consider using digital tools like apps that log your meals and physical activity to track your progress. Apps like **MyFitnessPal** or **Yazio** help you monitor your intake of specific nutrients and allow you to see trends over time, which can be incredibly motivating. Additionally, these tools often provide feedback and reminders, helping keep your goals at the forefront of your daily activities.

Celebrating Small Wins

Every small victory counts and deserves recognition on your journey to reducing inflammation through diet. Celebrating these milestones is vital as it helps build momentum and keeps your motivation high. This stress on celebrating small wins encourages you, making you feel motivated and eager to continue your health journey.

- Did you choose a salad over fries at lunch? That's a win.
- Managed to drink the recommended amount of water for a whole week? Another win.

These achievements, though small, are stepping stones toward your larger health goals. Acknowledging them reinforces your commitment and provides a psychological boost. Create a "success log" where you record these victories or share them with friends or in a support group. Seeing your progress laid out can be incredibly uplifting and spur you to maintain and build on these healthier habits.

Coping with Plateaus and Setbacks

It's natural to encounter plateaus or setbacks in your health journey. Encountering a weight loss stall or reverting to old eating habits is a common hurdle. During these times, adjusting your expectations and strategy is crucial. Adjust your goals to avoid any sense of discouragement. First, reassess your goals to ensure they're still realistic. It may be necessary to tweak your approach. Consider varying your diet more to renew your interest and nutrient intake or setting smaller, more achievable goals. Importantly, view these setbacks as learning opportunities. Analyze what led to the plateau or relapse—was it stress, unavailability of healthy food options, or simply boredom with your routine? Understanding these triggers enables you to develop strategies to overcome them in the future.

Staying Inspired

Keeping your motivation up can also come from external sources of inspiration. Follow health blogs, listen to podcasts about nutrition, or join online forums that focus on anti-inflammatory living. Engaging with content that educates and inspires can introduce new ideas and perspectives that boost your interest and commitment. For instance, subscribing to a newsletter from a trusted nutrition expert can provide you with a steady stream of fresh recipes and the latest research on diet and inflammation. Additionally, consider reading up on the latest scientific studies on anti-inflammatory diets and their benefits. Knowledge is power, and understanding your dietary choices' profound impact on your health can be a powerful motivator.

By integrating these strategies into your routine, you create a robust framework that supports sustained motivation. Whether it's through setting clear goals, celebrating every small success, learning from the setbacks, or seeking inspiration from the world around you, each step you take on this path is a building block toward a healthier, more vibrant you. Remember, the key to staying motivated is to recognize that each day presents a new opportunity to advance toward your ultimate health goals.

The Role of Community in Lifestyle Change

The journey can sometimes feel lonely or overwhelming when you start making significant changes to your diet and lifestyle, especially when aiming to reduce inflammation through natural remedies and healthier eating habits. It's often about more than just choosing different foods. It's about transforming your lifestyle, habits, and, sometimes, how you interact with others. The power of community comes into play during this transformative stage. Finding and engaging with support groups can be incredibly beneficial. These groups provide a platform for sharing experiences and tips, offering both emotional and practical support. Whether these are online forums focused on anti-inflammatory living or local groups that meet in person, they can become a crucial part of your support system.

For instance, online communities on platforms like Facebook or Reddit often have dedicated groups where members share their successes, challenges, and recipes. These platforms allow you to connect with people from all over the world, providing you with access to a wide array of experiences and advice. Moreover, these communities are accessible anytime, so you can find support and motivation whenever you need it, right at your fingertips. On the other hand, local support groups, often found through wellness centers or hospitals, provide the added benefit of face-to-face interaction. These meetings can sometimes include workshops or cooking demonstrations, which can be very beneficial for learning practical skills in a supportive environment.

Participating in community events is another excellent way to deepen your engagement with the anti-inflammatory lifestyle. Many communities offer health-related events like local farmers' markets, cooking classes, or health seminars. These events provide an opportunity to learn and meet others who are on a similar path, allowing for the exchange of ideas and building relationships with like-minded individuals. For example, a cooking class can teach you how to prepare anti-inflammatory meals while you interact with fellow attendees, which can provide insights into managing the challenges of maintaining such a lifestyle.

If finding an existing group that meets your needs proves challenging, consider starting your own. Taking the initiative can be a fulfilling way to meet others who share your interests and to actively contribute to spreading awareness about the benefits of an anti-inflammatory lifestyle. Starting a group does not have to be complicated. You can begin by setting up informal meet-ups at a local community center or via online platforms. The key is to create a welcoming environment where everyone feels comfortable sharing their experiences and advice. To attract members, you can use social media platforms, community bulletin boards, or local community newsletters to advertise your group. Planning the first few meetings with specific topics or guest speakers helps draw in participants who are looking for structured information and support.

Engaging with a community, whether by joining existing groups or starting your own, offers numerous benefits that can significantly enhance your journey toward a healthier lifestyle. It provides a sense of belonging and motivation, which can be crucial in maintaining long-term changes. Additionally, the shared experiences and collective knowledge found in these groups can empower you with new strategies and confidence to overcome challenges, making your transition to an anti-inflammatory diet both successful and enjoyable. As you continue to explore and integrate these community resources into your life, remember that each interaction and new connection is a step forward in your health journey and in fostering a broader understanding and adoption of healthier living.

Celebrating Your Successes: Milestones and Rewards

As you advance in your anti-inflammatory dietary journey, it's essential to recognize and celebrate the milestones you achieve along the way. These celebrations are not just about giving yourself a pat on the back—they are crucial psychological reinforcements that underscore your progress and solidify your commitment to a healthier lifestyle. Identifying these milestones can vary widely among individuals, depending on personal health goals and challenges. For some, it might be losing some weight or achieving a fitness goal like completing a 5K run. For others, significant milestones could include reducing their medication dosage under a doctor's supervision or going a certain period without a flare-up of inflammatory symptoms. Recognizing these achievements provides a tangible sense of progress and can be highly motivating.

When planning how to celebrate these milestones, it's very important to choose rewards that align with your health goals and enhance your wellness journey rather than contradict them. While an indulgent treat might seem tempting, consider opting for rewards that will support your ongoing commitment to an anti-inflammatory lifestyle. For instance, a day at a spa, investing in new workout gear or attending a healthy cooking class not only celebrates your achievements but also encourages your continued success. These rewards should feel like a personal treat, which also reinforces your healthy habits.

Sharing your successes plays a vital role in solidifying your achievements. By communicating your milestones with friends, family, or members of your support group, you enhance your feelings of accomplishment and inspire others to continue in their efforts or start on their health journeys. Sharing can be as simple as posting on your social media, participating in group discussions, or even just talking about your achievements with friends over coffee. These conversations can lead to positive feedback and encouragement, which bolster your motivation to maintain your anti-inflammatory lifestyle.

Incorporating reflective practices into your routine is another powerful tool for appreciating and understanding your health journey. Practices like journaling or meditation allow you to internalize your progress and reflect on the changes you've experienced. Journaling, for instance, can help you document not just your achievements but also the challenges you've faced, how you've overcome them, and how you feel physically and mentally. Over time, reviewing your journal entries can offer profound insights into the patterns and habits that contribute to your well-being. This reflection celebrates how far you've come and guides your future decisions. This practice also helps you adjust your approach, as needed, to continue progressing.

Through these practices—identifying milestones, planning appropriate rewards, sharing successes, and engaging in reflective activities—you create a cycle of positive reinforcement that celebrates your past achievements and propels you toward future ones. This approach turns each step of your health journey into an opportunity for celebration and growth, making the process enjoyable and sustainable in the long term. By recognizing and celebrating each success, you enhance your motivation and establish a lifestyle that continually supports your health and well-being. This dynamic process of celebration and reflection ensures that your journey toward reducing inflammation remains vibrant, rewarding, and tailored to your evolving health needs.

Adjusting Your Mindset for Health and Wellness

Adopting an anti-inflammatory lifestyle is as much about adjusting how you think about health and wellness as it is about changing what you eat. To make lasting changes, it's essential to shift your mindset from one of restriction to one focused on nourishment. Rather than viewing dietary changes as limiting, see them as opportunities to discover new foods and flavors and nourish your body in a way that supports its natural healing processes. This positive perspective helps maintain motivation and makes the dietary adjustments enjoyable rather than burdensome.

For many, negative self-talk can be a significant barrier to maintaining a healthy lifestyle. It's easy to berate oneself for slipping up or not making progress quickly enough. However, it's crucial to cultivate a kinder, more compassionate inner dialogue. Start by recognizing and challenging negative thoughts. For instance, if you catch yourself thinking, "I can't stick to this diet; it's too hard," try to reframe this thought to, "I'm finding some aspects of this diet challenging, but I'm learning and getting better every day." This shift alleviates unnecessary pressure and empowers you to continue making efforts without harsh self-judgment.

Embracing a holistic view of health is another vital aspect of adjusting your mindset. Health is a state of complete physical, mental, and social well-being and not solely the absence of disease or infirmity. An anti-inflammatory diet is an amazing tool for enhancing physical health. However, it's most effective when combined with other wellness practices like regular exercise, adequate sleep, and stress management. For instance, integrating mindfulness or yoga into your routine can significantly reduce stress levels, complementing your dietary efforts and promoting overall well-being. By adopting a more inclusive approach to health, you ensure that your efforts are balanced and sustainable.

Relapses in diet or lifestyle changes are expected and entirely normal. Treat them as learning opportunities instead of viewing them as failures. Each relapse can provide valuable insights into what triggers your old habits and how you can better manage those triggers in the future. For example, if you find yourself reverting to unhealthy eating habits during particularly stressful periods, this is an indicator that your current stress management strategies need strengthening. Consider incorporating more physical activity or practicing relaxation techniques to help you manage stress more effectively, which will, in turn, help you maintain your dietary changes. By learning from each relapse and making the necessary adjustments, you continually refine your approach to health, making your lifestyle changes more resilient and tailored to your unique needs.

Shifting your focus to nourishment, fostering positive self-talk, adopting a holistic approach to health, and learning from setbacks help to create a supportive framework for your anti-inflammatory lifestyle. These mindset adjustments are not just about changing what you eat; they're about transforming your relationship with your body and with your health. They foster a deeper appreciation for the relationship between your diet and your overall well-being, guiding you toward a harmonious, fulfilling lifestyle that nurtures both your body and mind. As you continue to integrate these mindset shifts into your daily life, you'll find that maintaining an anti-inflammatory lifestyle becomes more intuitive and rewarding, reflecting not just a diet change but a true enhancement of your overall quality of life.

Encouraging Family and Friends to Join You on Your Journey

When you embark on a path to healthier living through an anti-inflammatory diet, sharing this experience with family and friends not only enriches the journey but can also help cement your new habits. Convincing loved ones to join you, however, can sometimes be challenging. Here are some strategies for effectively communicating the benefits, involving them in activities, and managing any resistance you may encounter, all while setting a positive example through your actions.

Communicating Benefits Effectively

Explaining the benefits of an anti-inflammatory lifestyle to your family and friends is important, and doing so in an informative and non-confrontational way can make all the difference. Start by sharing your personal experiences and the positive changes you've noticed. Perhaps you've seen a significant decrease in joint pain, an improvement in your skin, or a boost in your energy levels. Personal stories are powerful and can pique interest more than general health advice. When discussing these benefits, focus on the positives—more energy, better health, delicious foods—rather than framing it as combating illness.

Additionally, be prepared with facts. Sometimes, loved ones may be more receptive when presented with information from credible sources. Share articles, books, or even snippets from documentaries that explain the science behind the anti-inflammatory diet and its benefits.

Involving Others in Activities

Involving family and friends in anti-inflammatory activities can be a fun and effective way to encourage them to embrace this lifestyle. One of the most engaging activities is cooking together. Plan a cooking night where you try out new anti-inflammatory recipes. Gatherings like these make meal prep enjoyable and educate participants about the ingredients and methods that reduce inflammation. Another idea is to organize regular outings that involve physical activity, which also plays a significant role in reducing inflammation. Whether it's a weekly family hike, a bike ride with friends, or a yoga session, these activities promote health and provide an opportunity to spend quality time together.

Dealing with Resistance

Resistance from loved ones can be one of the tougher aspects of transitioning to an anti-inflammatory lifestyle, especially when dietary changes challenge long-standing eating habits. If resistance arises, first ensure you genuinely listen to their concerns. Understanding their hesitations can help you address them more effectively. For instance, if a family member is worried about giving up certain foods they love, suggest modifications or alternatives that are healthier but still satisfying. It's also helpful to introduce changes gradually rather than expecting a complete overhaul overnight. Sometimes, all it takes is time for others to see the positive changes in you, which can naturally encourage them to try these changes themselves. If resistance persists, seek external support. Nutritionists, dietitians, or even local support groups can offer professional insights that may be more convincing.

Role Modeling

The most potent tool in your arsenal is to be a living example of the benefits of an anti-inflammatory lifestyle. You naturally inspire those around you by consistently adhering to your diet and showing tangible health improvements. Let your energy, vitality, and health speak for themselves. Often, seeing is believing, and when family and friends notice the positive changes in your life, their skepticism may turn into curiosity. Demonstrating that an anti-inflammatory lifestyle is not only feasible but also enjoyable and beneficial can motivate others to consider similar changes. Maintaining a positive and open attitude toward your lifestyle choices can encourage others to share your journey without feeling judged or pressured.

By effectively communicating the benefits, involving loved ones in fun and healthy activities, gracefully handling resistance, and leading by example, you enhance your own experience and potentially improve the health and well-being of those around you. Each of these strategies helps weave your anti-inflammatory lifestyle into the fabric of your social and family life, making it a shared journey of discovery and health.

As this chapter closes, we reflect on the importance of community and support in maintaining a health-focused lifestyle. Integrating an anti-inflammatory diet is an enriching experience when shared with others, offering mutual encouragement and deeper connections. As you move ahead, you will continue to explore practical ways to sustain and deepen these dietary and lifestyle changes, ensuring they remain enjoyable and beneficial in the long term.

Conclusion

As we reach the end of our journey together in *The Practical Anti-Inflammatory Diet Guide for Beginners*, it's helpful to look back and appreciate the ground we've covered. We've unraveled the complexities of inflammation, distinguishing between acute and chronic forms and understanding its profound impact on our health. We've explored how an anti-inflammatory diet is not just a means of managing symptoms but a pathway to enhanced overall well-being.

Throughout this guide, we've emphasized the importance of whole, unprocessed foods, a balanced intake of macronutrients, and the inclusion of diverse, colorful fruits and vegetables. We've learned that nuts, seeds, and healthy fats are not just tasty additions to our diet but are crucial in combating inflammation. Equally, we've recognized the need to reduce our intake of processed foods, refined sugars, and unhealthy fats.

However, managing inflammation extends beyond diet. Regular physical activity, effective stress management, adequate sleep, proper hydration, and the careful use of supplements form the pillars of a holistic anti-inflammatory lifestyle. Remember, the journey to reduce inflammation is all-embracing, incorporating multiple aspects of health and daily living.

This book has continually stressed the significance of personalization in your anti-inflammatory journey. There is no universal solution; what works wonderfully for one person might be less effective for another. I encourage you to listen closely to your body, experiment with your diet, and adjust your lifestyle in response to your unique health feedback. This personalized approach can be reassuring and also ensures that your strategies are effective and sustainable.

Staying informed is crucial. The field of nutrition and inflammation is ever-evolving, with new research and insights emerging regularly. Keep your curiosity alive and remain open to modifying your approach as you learn more about what best supports your health.

Embracing this new way of living may be challenging at times. It's normal to face hurdles and feel like reverting to old habits. However, remember to be patient with yourself. Celebrate each small victory, whether it's choosing a healthy meal over a fast-food option or simply opting for water instead of a sugary drink. Each positive choice is a step toward a healthier you.

Now, I urge you to take that first step. Whether it's swapping out a specific snack for a healthier option, setting a weekly goal for physical activity, or ensuring you are adequately hydrated throughout the day, start small and build from there. Set realistic and achievable goals and gradually incorporate more changes as you grow more comfortable with this new lifestyle.

Conclusion

Thank you for trusting me to guide you on this path to understanding and managing inflammation. You are not alone in this journey. For further information and support, I encourage you to explore online resources, join support groups, or consult nutrition professionals who can provide personalized guidance.

Remember, every step you take is a move toward a healthier, more vibrant life. Here's to making lasting changes that manage inflammation and enhance your overall well-being. Let's continue this journey together, learning, adapting, and thriving every step of the way.

With gratitude, I wish you the best for your health journey.

Bonus Chapter with Additional Recipes

This bonus chapter is provided to help you get started on your journey to an anti-inflammatory lifestyle. The recipes are for anti-inflammatory alternatives to a selection of comfort foods and one-pot dishes. One -pot dishes can be very handy when you are on a tight schedule. The list of recipes is below. Feel free to modify any of these recipes to fit your taste so that the anti-inflammatory meal feels like it was created for you.

List of Recipes for Comfort Foods

1. Oatmeal Banana Pancakes with Berry Compote (An alternative to Traditional Pancakes)
2. Whole Grain Veggie Pizza with Anti-Inflammatory Toppings
3. Baked or Air-Fried Anti-Inflammatory Chicken (An alternative to Fried Chicken)
4. Anti-Inflammatory Veggie Grilled Sandwich

5. Anti-Inflammatory Turkey or Veggie Burger (an alternative to Cheeseburger)
6. Cauliflower "Mac" and Cheese (an alternative to Mac and Cheese)
7. Nut-Free Cauliflower "Mac" and Cheese (an alternative to Mac and Cheese)
8. Baked Zucchini "Ziti" with Cashew Cheese (an alternative to Baked Ziti)
9. Baked Cauliflower Wings with Sweet Potato Fries (an alternative to Chicken Wings and Fries)
10. Zucchini Noodles with turkey meatballs and tomato sauce (an alternative to Spaghetti and Meatballs)

List of Recipes for One-Pot Dishes

1. Turmeric Lentil Soup
2. Quinoa and Vegetable Pilaf
3. Chickpea and Spinach Stew
4. Mexican Black Beans and Rice
5. Mediterranean Chickpeas and Rice
6. Caribbean Red Beans and Rice

Recipes: Anti-Inflammatory Comfort Foods

1. Oatmeal Banana Pancakes with Berry Compote

Here is the recipe for a healthier, anti-inflammatory alternative to traditional pancakes and syrup. This alternative uses whole, nutrient-dense ingredients that are lower in refined sugars and higher in fiber and antioxidants. Here's the recipe and explanation for the ingredient choices:

Ingredients:

For the Pancakes:

- 1 cup rolled oats (or oat flour for smoother texture)
- 2 ripe bananas
- 2 eggs
- 1/2 cup unsweetened almond milk (or use any plant-based milk)
- 1 teaspoon cinnamon
- 1 teaspoon baking powder (leavening agent)
- 1 teaspoon vanilla extract (flavor)
- Coconut oil or olive oil for cooking (healthy fats)

For the Berry Compote:

- 1 cup mixed berries (blueberries, strawberries, raspberries)
- 1–2 tablespoons water
- 1–2 teaspoons maple syrup or honey (optional for natural sweetness)

Instructions:

1. Prepare the Pancake Batter:

- Blend the rolled oats in a blender until they form a flour-like consistency (if using whole oats).
- In a mixing bowl, mash the bananas until smooth.
- Add eggs, almond milk, cinnamon, baking powder, and vanilla extract to the bananas and mix well.
- Stir in the oat flour until well combined. Allow the batter to sit for a few minutes to thicken.

2. Cook the Pancakes:

- Heat a non-stick skillet or griddle over medium heat, and use coconut or olive oil to lightly grease it.
- Pour 1/4 cup of batter onto the skillet for each pancake.
- Cook until bubbles form on the surface and the edges look set. Turn over and cook for another 1-2 minutes until golden brown.

3. Prepare the Berry Compote:

- In a small saucepan, combine mixed berries and water.
- Cook over medium heat, stirring occasionally, until the berries break down and the mixture thickens (about 5-7 minutes).
- If desired, add a small amount of maple syrup or honey for sweetness.

4. Serve:

- Stack the pancakes on a plate and top with warm berry compote.
- Optionally, add a dollop of Greek yogurt or a sprinkle of chopped nuts for added protein and healthy fats.

Ingredient Benefits:

- **Rolled Oats**: High in fiber, help regulate blood sugar and support heart health. Oats also contain antioxidants that have anti-inflammatory properties.
- **Bananas**: Provide natural sweetness, causing little to no

need for added sugars. They are rich in potassium and vitamin C, which can help reduce inflammation.
- **Eggs**: A good source of high-quality protein and contain essential vitamins and minerals.
- **Almond Milk**: A dairy-free option that is low in calories and often fortified with vitamins.
- **Cinnamon**: Contains anti-inflammatory and antioxidant compounds.
- **Mixed Berries**: Packed with vitamins, fiber, and antioxidants, they help fight inflammation and provide natural sweetness.

This alternative reduces refined sugars and unhealthy fats and includes ingredients known for their anti-inflammatory benefits. These pancakes will provide you with sustained energy and support overall health.

2. Whole Grain Veggie Pizza with Anti-Inflammatory Toppings

Here is a recipe for an anti-inflammatory pizza using whole grain crust. This pizza includes anti-inflammatory ingredients like vegetables, herbs, and healthy fats.

Ingredients:

For the Whole Grain Crust:

- 1 1/2 cups whole wheat flour
- 1/2 cup warm water
- 1 tablespoon olive oil
- 1 teaspoon honey or maple syrup
- 1 teaspoon active dry yeast

- 1/2 teaspoon salt

For the Toppings:

- 1/2 cup tomato sauce (select no added sugar, organic if possible)
- 1 cup dairy-free cheese (such as almond cheese, cashew cheese, or nutritional yeast-based cheese)
- 1 cup fresh spinach, roughly chopped
- 1/2 red bell pepper, thinly sliced
- 1/4 red onion, thinly sliced
- 1/2 cup cherry tomatoes, halved
- 1/4 cup black olives, sliced
- 1 teaspoon dried oregano
- 1 teaspoon dried basil
- 1 tablespoon olive oil (for drizzling)

Instructions:

1. Prepare the Whole Grain Crust:

- In a small bowl, dissolve the honey or maple syrup in warm water. Sprinkle the yeast over the water and let it sit for about 5 minutes until it becomes frothy.
- In a large bowl, mix the whole wheat flour and salt. Make a well in the center and add the yeast mixture and olive oil.
- Mix until the dough forms. Turn the dough out onto a lightly floured surface and knead for about 5–7 minutes until smooth and elastic.
- Put the dough in a lightly oiled bowl, cover it with a clean towel, and let the dough rise in a warm place for about 1 hour or until doubled in size.

2. Preheat the Oven:

- Preheat your oven to 450°F (230°C). Place a pizza stone or baking sheet in the oven to preheat it.

3. Roll Out the Dough:

- Once the dough has risen, punch it down and turn it out onto a lightly floured surface.
- Roll the dough out into a circle or rectangle, about 1/4 inch thick, depending on your preference.
- Place the rolled-out dough onto a piece of parchment paper.

4. Arrange the Pizza:

- Spread the tomato sauce evenly over the crust.
- Sprinkle the dairy-free cheese over the sauce.
- Add the spinach, red bell pepper, red onion, cherry tomatoes, and black olives.
- Sprinkle dried oregano and dried basil over the toppings.
- Drizzle with olive oil.

5. Bake the Pizza:

- Carefully transfer the parchment paper with the assembled pizza onto the preheated pizza stone or baking sheet.
- Bake for 12–15 minutes or until the crust is golden brown and the toppings are cooked.

6. Serve:

- Allow the pizza to cool for a few minutes before you slice and serve.

Ingredient Benefits:

- **Whole Wheat Flour**: Provides more fiber, vitamins, and minerals compared to refined flour, which helps stabilize blood sugar levels and reduce inflammation.
- **Olive Oil**: Rich in monounsaturated fats and antioxidants, which have anti-inflammatory properties.
- **Tomato Sauce**: Tomatoes are rich in lycopene, an antioxidant that helps reduce inflammation.
- **Dairy-Free Cheese**: Avoids the inflammatory effects of dairy for those who are sensitive to it.
- **Spinach**: High in vitamins A, C, and K and antioxidants, which help fight inflammation.
- **Red Bell Pepper**: Contains vitamins A and C, which are powerful antioxidants that help reduce inflammation.
- **Red Onion**: Contains quercetin, an antioxidant with anti-inflammatory effects.
- **Cherry Tomatoes**: Rich in lycopene, an antioxidant that helps reduce inflammation.
- **Black Olives**: Provide healthy fats and antioxidants that support heart health and reduce inflammation.
- **Herbs (Oregano, Basil)**: Provide antioxidants and anti-inflammatory properties, enhancing the flavor and health benefits of the pizza.

This whole-grain veggie pizza is a delicious and nutritious alternative to traditional pizza.

3. Baked or Air-Fried Anti-Inflammatory Chicken

Here is a recipe that provides the same satisfying crunch and flavor of fried chicken without the inflammatory effects of traditional frying:

Ingredients:

- 4 boneless, skinless chicken breasts or thighs
- 1 cup whole wheat flour or almond flour
- 1 cup whole wheat breadcrumbs or crushed whole grain crackers
- 1 teaspoon turmeric
- 1 teaspoon garlic powder
- 1 teaspoon paprika
- 1 teaspoon black pepper
- 1 teaspoon dried oregano
- 1 teaspoon sea salt
- 1 cup unsweetened almond milk or low-fat buttermilk
- 2 tablespoons olive oil or avocado oil (if using an oven)

Instructions:

1. **Preheat your oven or air fryer**:

- For oven: Preheat to 400°F (200°C).
- For air fryer: Preheat to 375°F (190°C) if your model requires preheating.

2. Prepare the coating:

- In a shallow dish, combine the flour, breadcrumbs, turmeric, garlic powder, paprika, black pepper, oregano, and salt.

3. Dip for the chicken:

- Pour the almond milk or buttermilk into another shallow dish.
- Dip each chicken piece into the milk. Coat it thoroughly in the flour mixture.

4. For Oven:

- Place the coated chicken pieces on a baking sheet lined with parchment paper.
- Drizzle the olive oil or avocado oil evenly over the chicken.
- Bake in the preheated oven for 25-30 minutes or until the chicken is golden brown and cooked through. Flip the chicken halfway through baking for even crispiness.

5. For Air Fryer:

- Place the coated chicken pieces in the air fryer basket in a single layer.
- Cook for 20-25 minutes, flipping halfway through, until the chicken is crispy and cooked through.

6. Serve:

- Enjoy your baked or air-fried chicken with a side of anti-inflammatory vegetables like steamed broccoli or a fresh salad.

Tips:

- **Marinate the Chicken**: Marinate the chicken in almond milk or buttermilk for a few hours for extra flavor and tenderness before coating.
- **Spice Variations**: Feel free to adjust the spices to your taste. Adding cayenne pepper can give a spicy kick, while herbs like rosemary and thyme can add different flavors.

This alternative to fried chicken is healthier and helps reduce inflammation while still giving you that delicious crunch you crave.

Ingredient Benefits:

- **Boneless, Skinless Chicken Breasts or Thighs:** Chicken is a lean source of protein, essential for muscle repair and overall health. It provides important nutrients like B vitamins and minerals, while the skinless option reduces saturated fat intake, which is beneficial for reducing inflammation.
- **Whole Wheat Flour or Almond Flour:** Whole wheat flour is rich in fiber and nutrients, promoting digestive health and stabilizing blood sugar levels, which helps reduce inflammation. Almond flour is a gluten-free option that is high in healthy fats, fiber, and vitamin E, providing antioxidant and anti-inflammatory benefits.

- **Whole Wheat Breadcrumbs or Crushed Whole Grain Crackers:** These add a crunchy texture while providing fiber and nutrients that support digestive health. Whole grains are associated with lower levels of inflammation and improved heart health.
- **Turmeric:** Contains curcumin, a powerful anti-inflammatory and antioxidant compound that helps reduce chronic inflammation and supports overall health.
- **Garlic Powder:** Has sulfur compounds that have potent anti-inflammatory and immune-boosting properties, helping to fight inflammation and reduce the risk of chronic diseases.
- **Paprika:** Adds flavor and contains antioxidants like capsaicin, which has anti-inflammatory properties and may help reduce pain and inflammation.
- **Black Pepper:** Contains piperine, which enhances the absorption of curcumin from turmeric, making it more effective in reducing inflammation. It also has its own anti-inflammatory and antioxidant properties.
- **Dried Oregano:** Rich in antioxidants and has anti-inflammatory properties, contributing to the reduction of oxidative stress and supporting immune health.
- **Sea Salt:** When used in moderation, sea salt provides essential minerals and helps balance electrolytes, supporting overall health.
- **Unsweetened Almond Milk or Low-Fat Buttermilk:** Almond milk is a dairy-free alternative that provides vitamin E and healthy fats, which have anti-inflammatory properties. Low-fat buttermilk is rich in probiotics and calcium, promoting gut health and reducing inflammation.
- **Olive Oil or Avocado Oil:** Both oils are rich in healthy monounsaturated fats and antioxidants. Olive oil is well-

known for its anti-inflammatory effects, while avocado oil is rich in vitamin E and supports heart health.

4. Anti-Inflammatory Veggie Grilled Sandwich

Here is a recipe for an anti-inflammatory alternative to a traditional grilled cheese sandwich using nutrient-dense, whole-food ingredients. Instead of processed cheese and refined bread, this alternative uses whole grain or gluten-free bread and dairy-free cheese, and it adds anti-inflammatory vegetables.

Ingredients:

- 2 slices whole grain or gluten-free bread
- 1/2 avocado, mashed
- 1/2 cup dairy-free cheese (such as almond cheese, cashew cheese, or nutritional yeast-based cheese)
- 1/2 cup fresh spinach or kale
- 1/2 roasted red bell pepper, sliced
- 1/4 cup thinly sliced red onion
- 1 tablespoon olive oil or avocado oil

Instructions:

1. Prepare the Ingredients:

- If using roasted red bell peppers, you can either roast them yourself by placing them in the oven at 400°F (200°C) until the skin is charred, then peeling off the skin, or use store-bought roasted peppers.
- Wash and dry the spinach or kale.

2. Arrange the Sandwich:

- Spread the mashed avocado evenly on one side of each slice of bread.
- Layer the dairy-free cheese, fresh spinach or kale, roasted red bell pepper slices, and thinly sliced red onion on one slice of bread.
- Top with the other slice of bread, avocado side down, to form a sandwich.

3. Grill the Sandwich:

- Heat the olive oil or avocado oil in a skillet over medium heat.
- Place the sandwich in the skillet and cook until the bread is golden brown and crispy, about 3–4 minutes per side. Press down gently with a spatula to help melt the cheese and ensure even grilling.
- If needed, cover the skillet with a lid for a few minutes to help melt the cheese completely.

4. Serve:

- Cut the sandwich in half and serve hot.

Ingredient Benefits:

- **Whole Grain or Gluten-Free Bread**: Provides fiber, vitamins, and minerals. Whole grains help reduce inflammation by stabilizing blood sugar levels and supporting gut health.

- **Avocado**: Rich in healthy monounsaturated fats, vitamins, and antioxidants, which have anti-inflammatory properties.
- **Dairy-Free Cheese**: Made from nuts or other plant-based ingredients, these cheeses are free from the inflammatory compounds found in dairy. Nutritional yeast-based cheese is also rich in B vitamins and has a cheesy flavor.
- **Spinach or Kale**: These leafy greens are packed with vitamins A, C, and K, as well as antioxidants and anti-inflammatory compounds.
- **Roasted Red Bell Pepper**: High in vitamins A and C, which are powerful antioxidants that help reduce inflammation.
- **Red Onion**: Contains quercetin, an antioxidant that has anti-inflammatory effects.
- **Olive Oil or Avocado Oil**: Both oils are rich in healthy fats and antioxidants that support heart health and reduce inflammation.

This veggie grilled sandwich provides a delicious and nutritious alternative to traditional grilled cheese.

5. Anti-Inflammatory Turkey or Veggie Burger

Here is a recipe for a healthier, anti-inflammatory alternative to a cheeseburger. You can make a delicious and nutritious turkey or veggie burger with anti-inflammatory ingredients.

Ingredients:

For the Turkey Burgers:

- 1 lb. ground turkey (preferably lean)

- 1/2 cup finely chopped onions
- 2 cloves garlic, minced
- 1 teaspoon turmeric
- 1 teaspoon cumin
- 1/2 teaspoon black pepper
- 1/2 teaspoon sea salt
- 1/4 cup finely chopped parsley or cilantro
- 1 tablespoon olive oil (for cooking)

For the Veggie Burger:

- 1 can (15 oz) black beans or chickpeas, drained and rinsed
- 1/2 cup finely chopped onions
- 1/2 cup grated carrots or zucchini
- 2 cloves garlic, minced
- 1 teaspoon turmeric
- 1 teaspoon cumin
- 1/2 teaspoon black pepper
- 1/2 teaspoon sea salt
- 1/4 cup finely chopped parsley or cilantro
- 1/2 cup whole wheat breadcrumbs or oat flour
- 1 tablespoon olive oil (for cooking)

Toppings:

- Sliced avocado
- Fresh spinach or arugula
- Tomato slices
- Red onion slices
- Anti-inflammatory cheese option (such as goat cheese or dairy-free cheese)
- Whole grain buns or lettuce wrap

Instructions:

1. Prepare the Burger Patties:

- **For Turkey Burgers:** In a large bowl, combine ground turkey, onions, garlic, turmeric, cumin, black pepper, sea salt, and parsley/cilantro. Mix well and form into patties. Expect to form up to 4 patties from this mixture.
- **For Veggie Burgers:** In a large bowl, mash the beans or chickpeas until mostly smooth. Add onions, grated carrots/zucchini, garlic, turmeric, cumin, black pepper, sea salt, parsley/cilantro, and breadcrumbs/oat flour. Mix well and form into patties. Expect to form up to 4 patties.

2. Cook the Patties:

- Heat olive oil in a skillet over medium heat.
- Cook the patties for about 5-6 minutes on each side or until they are cooked through (for turkey) or crispy on the outside (for veggie).

3. Arrange the Burger:

- Place each cooked patty on a whole-grain bun or lettuce wrap.
- Top with sliced avocado, fresh spinach or arugula, tomato slices, red onion slices, and your choice of anti-inflammatory cheese.

4. Serve:

- Enjoy your anti-inflammatory burger with a side of sweet potato fries or a fresh salad.

Tips:

- **Marinate the Patties**: For extra flavor, let the turkey or veggie patties sit for 30 minutes before cooking.
- **Spice Variations**: Adjust spices to your preference. Adding a pinch of cayenne pepper can add a spicy kick, while herbs like rosemary and thyme can offer different flavors.
- **Condiments**: Use anti-inflammatory condiments like hummus, guacamole, or mustard instead of ketchup and mayo.

Ingredient Benefits:

For the Turkey Burgers:

- **Ground Turkey**: Lean protein source that is lower in saturated fats compared to red meat, helping to reduce inflammation.
- **Onions**: High in antioxidants like quercetin, which have anti-inflammatory effects.
- **Garlic**: Contains sulfur compounds that have powerful anti-inflammatory and immune-boosting properties.
- **Turmeric**: Contains curcumin, a potent anti-inflammatory compound that helps reduce chronic inflammation.
- **Cumin**: Rich in antioxidants and anti-inflammatory compounds.

- **Black Pepper**: Contains piperine, which enhances the absorption of curcumin from turmeric.
- **Sea Salt**: Used in moderation, it provides essential minerals and enhances flavor.
- **Parsley or Cilantro**: Rich in vitamins A, C, and K and has antioxidant and anti-inflammatory properties.
- **Olive Oil:** Contains healthy monounsaturated fats and antioxidants that have anti-inflammatory effects.

For the Veggie Burger:

- **Black Beans or Chickpeas**: High in fiber, protein, and antioxidants, helping to reduce inflammation and support overall health.
- **Onions**: High in antioxidants like quercetin, which have anti-inflammatory effects.
- **Carrots or Zucchini**: Rich in vitamins A and C and antioxidants that support overall health and reduce inflammation.
- **Garlic**: Contains sulfur compounds that have powerful anti-inflammatory and immune-boosting properties.
- **Turmeric**: Contains curcumin, a potent anti-inflammatory compound that helps reduce chronic inflammation.
- **Cumin**: Rich in antioxidants and anti-inflammatory compounds.
- **Black Pepper**: Contains piperine, which enhances the absorption of curcumin from turmeric.
- **Sea Salt**: Used in moderation, it provides essential minerals and enhances flavor.
- **Parsley or Cilantro**: Rich in vitamins A, C, and K and has antioxidant and anti-inflammatory properties.

- **Whole Wheat Breadcrumbs or Oat Flour**: Adds fiber and helps bind the ingredients together, supporting digestive health.
- **Olive Oil**: Contains healthy monounsaturated fats and antioxidants that have anti-inflammatory effects.

For the Toppings:

- **Avocado Slices**: Rich in monounsaturated fats, fiber, and antioxidants, which help reduce inflammation.
- **Fresh Spinach or Arugula**: High in vitamins A, C, and K and antioxidants that support overall health and reduce inflammation.
- **Tomato Slices**: Rich in lycopene, an antioxidant that helps reduce inflammation.
- **Red Onion Slices**: Contains quercetin, an antioxidant with anti-inflammatory effects.
- **Whole Grain Buns or Lettuce Wrap**: Whole grain buns provide fiber and nutrients, while lettuce wraps are a low-carb option rich in vitamins and antioxidants.

The turkey or veggie alternative provides the satisfaction of a traditional cheeseburger while avoiding the inflammatory effects.

6. Cauliflower "Mac" and Cheese

Here is a recipe for an alternative to traditional macaroni and cheese. This dish uses cauliflower instead of pasta and a creamy, dairy-free cheese sauce made from cashews and nutritional yeast.

Ingredients:

For the Cauliflower "Mac":

- 1 large head of cauliflower, cut into florets
- 1 tablespoon olive oil
- Salt and pepper to taste

For the Cheese Sauce:

- 1 cup raw cashews (soaked in hot water for 15 minutes)
- 1/2 cup unsweetened almond milk (or use any plant-based milk)
- 1/4 cup nutritional yeast
- 1 tablespoon lemon juice (adds tanginess and vitamin C)
- 1 teaspoon garlic powder
- 1 teaspoon onion powder
- 1 teaspoon turmeric (adds color)
- 1/2 teaspoon mustard powder (enhances cheesy flavor)
- Salt and pepper to taste

Optional Toppings:

- 1/4 cup breadcrumbs or ground almonds (for a crunchy topping, if desired)
- 1 tablespoon olive oil (for drizzling on top)

Instructions:

1. Prepare the Cauliflower:

- Preheat your oven to 400°F (200°C).

- Toss the cauliflower florets together with olive oil, salt, and pepper.
- Spread the florets on a baking sheet. Roast for 20-25 minutes until tender and slightly golden.

2. Make the Cheese Sauce:

- Drain the soaked cashews and add them to a blender or food processor.
- Add almond milk, nutritional yeast, lemon juice, garlic powder, onion powder, turmeric, mustard powder, salt and pepper.
- Blend until the mixture is smooth and creamy. Adjust seasoning to taste.

3. Arrange the Ingredients for the Dish:

- Place the roasted cauliflower florets in a large mixing bowl.
- Pour the cheese sauce over the cauliflower and toss until evenly coated.

4. Bake (Optional):

- Transfer the cauliflower and cheese sauce mixture to a baking dish.
- If using, sprinkle breadcrumbs or ground almonds on top and drizzle with olive oil.
- Bake at 400°F (200°C) for 10-15 minutes until the topping is golden and crispy.

5. Serve:

- Enjoy your cauliflower "mac" and cheese as a delicious, anti-inflammatory alternative to traditional macaroni and cheese.

Ingredient Benefits:

- **Cauliflower**: A nutrient-dense vegetable that provides a low-carb alternative to pasta. It's high in vitamins C and K, fiber, and antioxidants, which can help reduce inflammation.
- **Cashews**: These nuts provide a creamy texture for the sauce and are rich in healthy fats, protein, and minerals like magnesium, which is known for its anti-inflammatory properties.
- **Nutritional Yeast**: A vegan-friendly ingredient that adds a cheesy flavor without dairy. It's also a great source of B vitamins and antioxidants.
- **Almond Milk**: A dairy-free base that is low in calories and often fortified with vitamins.
- **Spices (Turmeric, Garlic Powder, Onion Powder, Mustard Powder)**: These add flavor and have anti-inflammatory properties. Turmeric, in particular, contains curcumin, which is a powerful anti-inflammatory compound.
- **Olive Oil**: A source of healthy monounsaturated fats and antioxidants that can help reduce inflammation.

This cauliflower "mac" and cheese offers a creamy, cheesy experience and excludes dairy and refined carbs. It's a delicious and nutritious alternative.

7. Nut-Free Cauliflower "Mac" and Cheese

If you have a nut allergy or intolerance, you can still enjoy a delicious and creamy cauliflower "mac" and cheese by using seeds or other nut-free alternatives. Here is a nut-free version of the recipe, with substitutions and explanations of the chosen ingredients:

Ingredients:

For the Cauliflower "Mac":

- 1 large head of cauliflower, cut into florets (low-carb, high in vitamins and fiber)
- 1 tablespoon olive oil (healthy fat)
- Salt and pepper to taste

For the Cheese Sauce:

- 1 cup sunflower seeds (soaked in hot water for 15 minutes) (creamy texture and healthy fats without nuts)
- 1/2 cup unsweetened oat milk (or any plant-based milk) (dairy-free base)
- 1/4 cup nutritional yeast (provides a cheesy flavor and is rich in B vitamins)
- 1 tablespoon lemon juice (adds tanginess and vitamin C)
- 1 teaspoon garlic powder (anti-inflammatory properties)
- 1 teaspoon onion powder (flavor and anti-inflammatory properties)
- 1 teaspoon turmeric (adds color and anti-inflammatory benefits)
- 1/2 teaspoon mustard powder (enhances cheesy flavor)
- Salt and pepper to taste

Optional Toppings:

- 1/4 cup breadcrumbs or ground sunflower seeds (for a crunchy topping, if desired)
- 1 tablespoon olive oil (for drizzling on top)

Instructions:

1. Prepare the Cauliflower:

- Preheat your oven to 400°F (200°C).
- Toss the cauliflower florets together with olive oil, salt, and pepper.
- Spread the florets on a baking sheet. Roast for 20–25 minutes until tender and slightly golden.

2. Make the Cheese Sauce:

- Drain the soaked sunflower seeds and add them to a blender or food processor.
- Add oat milk, nutritional yeast, lemon juice, garlic powder, onion powder, turmeric, mustard powder, salt, and pepper.
- Blend until the mixture is smooth and creamy. Adjust seasoning to taste.

3. Arrange the Ingredients for the Dish:

- Place the roasted cauliflower florets in a large mixing bowl.
- Pour the cheese sauce over the cauliflower and toss until evenly coated.

4. Bake (Optional):

- Transfer the cauliflower and cheese sauce mixture to a baking dish.
- If using, sprinkle breadcrumbs or ground sunflower seeds on top and drizzle with olive oil.
- Bake at 400°F (200°C) for 10–15 minutes until the topping is golden and crispy.

5. Serve:

- Enjoy your nut-free cauliflower "mac" and cheese as a delicious, anti-inflammatory alternative to traditional macaroni and cheese.

Ingredient Benefits:

- **Sunflower Seeds**: These seeds provide a creamy texture for the sauce and are rich in healthy fats, protein, and minerals like magnesium, which is known for its anti-inflammatory properties. They are a great nut-free alternative for those with allergies.
- **Oat Milk**: A dairy-free base that is low in calories and often fortified with vitamins. It is a suitable alternative for those with nut allergies.
- **Nutritional Yeast**: A vegan-friendly ingredient that adds a cheesy flavor without dairy. It's also a great source of B vitamins and antioxidants.
- **Spices (Turmeric, Garlic Powder, Onion Powder, Mustard Powder)**: These add flavor and have anti-inflammatory properties. Turmeric, in particular, contains curcumin, which is a powerful anti-inflammatory

compound.
- **Olive Oil**: A source of healthy monounsaturated fats and antioxidants that can help reduce inflammation.

By using sunflower seeds and oat milk, you can create a nut-free version of cauliflower "mac" and cheese that is creamy and delicious. This alternative ensures that those with nut allergies or intolerances can still enjoy a comforting, anti-inflammatory meal.

8. Baked Zucchini "Ziti" with Cashew Cheese

Here is a recipe for creating an anti-inflammatory alternative to baked ziti using whole, nutrient-dense ingredients and avoiding common inflammatory triggers such as refined pasta and cheese.

Ingredients:

For the Zucchini "Ziti":

- 4–5 large zucchinis, sliced into thin, long strips (or use a spiralizer for zoodles)
- 1 tablespoon olive oil
- Salt and pepper to taste

For the Tomato Sauce:

- 1 tablespoon olive oil
- 1 onion, finely chopped
- 3 cloves garlic, minced
- 1 can (28 oz) crushed tomatoes
- 1 teaspoon dried oregano
- 1 teaspoon dried basil

- 1/2 teaspoon red pepper flakes (optional, if you wish for a spicy kick)
- Salt and pepper to taste

For the Cashew Cheese:

- 1 cup raw cashews (soaked in hot water for 15 minutes)
- 1/2 cup unsweetened almond milk (or use any plant-based milk)
- 1/4 cup nutritional yeast
- 1 tablespoon lemon juice
- 1 teaspoon garlic powder
- 1 teaspoon onion powder
- Salt and pepper to taste

Instructions:

1. Prepare the Zucchini:

- Preheat your oven to 375°F (190°C).
- Slice the zucchini into thin, long strips using a mandoline or a knife. Alternatively, use a spiralizer to create zoodles.
- Lightly salt the zucchini strips and let them sit for about 10 minutes to draw out excess moisture. Pat dry with paper towels.

2. Make the Tomato Sauce:

- Heat olive oil over medium heat in a large saucepan.
- Add chopped onion and cook until translucent, about 5 minutes.
- Add minced garlic. Cook for another minute until fragrant.

- Put in the crushed tomatoes, dried oregano, dried basil, red pepper flakes (optional), salt, and pepper.
- Simmer the sauce for about 15–20 minutes, stirring occasionally.

3. Make the Cashew Cheese:

- Drain the soaked cashews. Add them to a blender or food processor.
- Add almond milk, nutritional yeast, lemon juice, garlic powder, onion powder, salt, and pepper.
- Blend until the mixture is smooth and creamy. Adjust seasoning to taste.

4. Arrange the Ingredients for the Dish:

- Spread a thin layer of tomato sauce on the bottom of a baking dish.
- Layer half of the zucchini strips over the sauce.
- Spread half of the cashew cheese over the zucchini.
- Repeat with another layer of tomato sauce, zucchini strips, and the remaining cashew cheese.

5. Bake:

- Cover the baking dish with foil, and then bake it in the preheated oven for 20 minutes.
- Remove the foil and bake for an additional 10-15 minutes or until the top is lightly browned and bubbly.

6. Serve:

- Let the baked zucchini "ziti" cool for a few minutes before serving.
- Garnish with fresh basil or parsley if desired.

Ingredient Benefits:

- **Zucchini**: Provides a low-carb alternative to pasta, rich in vitamins A and C and high in fiber and antioxidants, which help reduce inflammation.
- **Olive Oil**: Contains healthy monounsaturated fats and antioxidants that have anti-inflammatory effects.
- **Onion and Garlic**: Both have anti-inflammatory and antioxidant properties, adding flavor and health benefits to the sauce.
- **Crushed Tomatoes**: High in antioxidants like lycopene, which help reduce inflammation.
- **Cashews**: Provide a creamy texture for the cheese sauce and are rich in healthy fats, protein, and minerals like magnesium, which have anti-inflammatory properties.
- **Nutritional Yeast**: Adds a cheesy flavor without dairy and is a good source of B vitamins and antioxidants.

This alternative to baked ziti offers a comforting, cheesy experience with ingredients that support an anti-inflammatory diet, providing health benefits without sacrificing flavor.

9. Baked Cauliflower Wings with Sweet Potato Fries

Here is a recipe for an anti-inflammatory alternative to traditional chicken wings and fries. This combination uses nutrient-dense, anti-inflammatory ingredients while still providing a satisfying, flavorful meal.

Ingredients:

For the Cauliflower Wings:

- 1 large head of cauliflower, cut into bite-sized florets
- 1/2 cup chickpea flour (or any gluten-free flour)
- 1/2 cup water (to make the batter)
- 1 teaspoon garlic powder
- 1 teaspoon onion powder
- 1/2 teaspoon paprika (adds smoky flavor)
- 1/2 teaspoon salt
- 1/4 teaspoon black pepper
- 1 cup hot sauce (look for one with simple ingredients and no added sugars)
- 1 tablespoon olive oil

For the Sweet Potato Fries:

- 2 large sweet potatoes, cut into fries
- 2 tablespoons olive oil
- 1 teaspoon smoked paprika
- 1/2 teaspoon garlic powder
- 1/2 teaspoon salt
- 1/4 teaspoon black pepper

Instructions:

1. Prepare the Cauliflower Wings:

1. Preheat your oven to 450°F (230°C).
2. In a large bowl, whisk together the chickpea flour, water, garlic powder, onion powder, paprika, salt, and black pepper to make a batter.
3. Dip each cauliflower floret into the batter, ensuring it is well coated. Shake off any excess batter.
4. Put the coated florets on a baking sheet lined with parchment paper.
5. Bake in the preheated oven for 20–25 minutes until the cauliflower is tender and the coating is crispy.
6. In a separate bowl, mix the hot sauce with olive oil. Toss the baked cauliflower florets in the sauce mixture.
7. Return the coated cauliflower wings to the oven and bake for an additional 10 minutes.

2. Prepare the Sweet Potato Fries:

1. While the cauliflower wings are baking, preheat another oven to 425°F (220°C) (or use the same oven after the wings are done).
2. Toss the sweet potato fries with olive oil, smoked paprika, garlic powder, salt, and black pepper in a large bowl.
3. Spread the fries in a single layer on a baking sheet lined with parchment paper.
4. Bake for 25–30 minutes, flipping halfway through, until the fries are crispy and golden brown.

3. Serve:

1. Serve the baked cauliflower wings with a side of sweet potato fries.
2. Optionally, provide dipping sauces like a homemade yogurt-based ranch or a tahini dip for added flavor and nutrition.

Ingredient Benefits:

- **Cauliflower**: A nutrient-dense vegetable rich in vitamins C and K, fiber, and antioxidants, which help reduce inflammation.
- **Chickpea Flour**: High in protein and fiber, this gluten-free flour provides a nutritious base for the batter and supports digestive health.
- **Olive Oil**: Contains healthy monounsaturated fats and antioxidants that have anti-inflammatory effects.
- **Sweet Potatoes**: High in vitamins A and C, fiber, and antioxidants like beta-carotene, which help reduce inflammation and support overall health.
- **Spices (Garlic Powder, Onion Powder, Paprika)**: These spices not only add flavor but also have anti-inflammatory properties, enhancing the health benefits of the dish.
- **Hot Sauce**: When choosing a hot sauce with simple, natural ingredients, it can add flavor without adding inflammatory additives.

This alternative to chicken wings and fries offers a satisfying and flavorful meal.

10. Zucchini Noodles with Turkey Meatballs and Tomato Sauce

Here is a recipe for an anti-inflammatory alternative to traditional spaghetti and meatballs, using whole, nutrient-dense ingredients while avoiding common inflammatory triggers such as refined pasta, red meat, and processed sauces.

Ingredients:

For the Zucchini Noodles:

- 4–5 large zucchinis, spiralized into noodles (zoodles)
- 1 tablespoon olive oil
- Salt and pepper to taste

For the Turkey Meatballs:

- 1 lb. ground turkey
- 1/4 cup finely chopped onions (flavor and anti-inflammatory properties)
- 2 cloves garlic, minced
- 1/4 cup whole wheat breadcrumbs (or gluten-free breadcrumbs if needed)
- 1/4 cup chopped fresh parsley
- 1 egg (binding agent and protein source)
- 1 teaspoon dried oregano
- 1 teaspoon dried basil
- 1/2 teaspoon salt
- 1/2 teaspoon black pepper

For the Tomato Sauce:

- 1 tablespoon olive oil
- 1 onion, finely chopped
- 3 cloves garlic, minced
- 1 can (28 oz) crushed tomatoes
- 1 teaspoon dried oregano
- 1 teaspoon dried basil
- 1/2 teaspoon red pepper flakes (optional, if you wish for a spicy kick)
- Salt and pepper to taste

Instructions:

1. Prepare the Zucchini Noodles:

- Spiralize the zucchini into noodles using a spiralizer.
- Lightly salt the zucchini noodles and let them sit for about 10 minutes to draw out excess moisture. Pat dry with paper towels.
- Heat olive oil in a large skillet over medium heat.
- Sauté the zucchini noodles for 3–5 minutes until just tender. Season with salt and pepper to taste. Set aside.

2. Make the Turkey Meatballs:

- Preheat your oven to 375°F (190°C).
- In a large bowl, combine ground turkey, chopped onions, minced garlic, breadcrumbs, chopped parsley, egg, dried oregano, dried basil, salt, and black pepper.
- Mix well and form into small meatballs (about 1 inch in diameter).

- Place the meatballs on a baking sheet lined with parchment paper.
- Bake in the preheated oven for 20–25 minutes or until cooked through and golden brown.

3. Make the Tomato Sauce:

- Heat olive oil in a large saucepan over medium heat.
- Add chopped onion and cook until translucent, about 5 minutes.
- Add minced garlic, then cook for another minute until fragrant.
- Put in the crushed tomatoes, dried oregano, dried basil, red pepper flakes (optional), salt, and pepper.
- Simmer the sauce for about 15–20 minutes, stirring occasionally.

4. Assemble the Dish:

- Add the baked turkey meatballs to the tomato sauce and let them simmer for a few minutes to absorb the flavors.
- Serve the meatballs and sauce over the sautéed zucchini noodles.

5. Serve:

- Garnish with fresh basil or parsley if desired.

Ingredient Benefits:

- **Zucchini**: Provides a low-carb alternative to pasta, rich in vitamins A and C and high in fiber and antioxidants, which help reduce inflammation.
- **Turkey**: A lean protein source that is lower in saturated fats compared to red meat, reducing the risk of inflammation.
- **Olive Oil**: Contains healthy monounsaturated fats and antioxidants that have anti-inflammatory effects.
- **Onion and Garlic**: Both have anti-inflammatory and antioxidant properties, adding flavor and health benefits to the dish.
- **Crushed Tomatoes**: High in antioxidants like lycopene, which help reduce inflammation.
- **Herbs (Oregano, Basil, Parsley)**: These herbs provide antioxidants and anti-inflammatory properties, enhancing the flavor and health benefits of the meal.

This alternative to spaghetti and meatballs provides a satisfying and flavorful meal and offers many health benefits while keeping the dish delicious. You may also try using whole-grain spaghetti noodles instead of zoodles.

Recipes: One-Pot Dishes

Here are a few anti-inflammatory one-pot dishes that are easy to make, packed with nutrients, and delicious. These recipes use ingredients known for their anti-inflammatory properties and are designed to be simple and convenient.

1. Turmeric Lentil Soup

Ingredients:

- 1 cup red lentils, rinsed
- 1 tablespoon olive oil
- 1 onion, finely chopped
- 2 cloves garlic, minced
- 1 tablespoon fresh ginger, minced
- 2 carrots, diced
- 2 celery stalks, diced
- 1 teaspoon ground turmeric
- 1 teaspoon ground cumin
- 1/2 teaspoon ground coriander
- 1/2 teaspoon paprika
- 1 can (14.5 oz) diced tomatoes
- 4 cups vegetable broth
- 1 can (14.5 oz) coconut milk
- Salt and pepper to taste
- Fresh cilantro, chopped (for garnish)
- Lemon wedges (for serving)

Instructions:

1. In a large pot, heat the olive oil over medium heat.
2. Add the onion, garlic, and ginger. Sauté until fragrant and the onion is translucent.
3. Add the carrots and celery and cook for another 5 minutes.
4. Stir in the turmeric, cumin, coriander, and paprika. Cook for 1 minute until the spices are fragrant.
5. Add the lentils, diced tomatoes, vegetable broth, and coconut milk. Bring to a boil.

6. Reduce the heat and let it simmer for 25–30 minutes or until the lentils and vegetables are tender.
7. Season with salt and pepper to taste.
8. Serve hot, garnished with fresh cilantro and lemon wedges.

Ingredient Benefits:

- **Red Lentils**: High in fiber and protein, support digestive health, and help stabilize blood sugar levels.
- **Olive Oil**: Contains healthy fats and antioxidants that reduce inflammation.
- **Onion and Garlic**: Rich in antioxidants and sulfur compounds that have anti-inflammatory and immune-boosting properties.
- **Ginger**: Contains gingerol, which has powerful anti-inflammatory and antioxidant effects.
- **Carrots and Celery**: Rich in vitamins, minerals, and antioxidants that support overall health and reduce inflammation.
- **Turmeric**: Contains curcumin, a powerful anti-inflammatory compound.
- **Cumin and Coriander**: Provide antioxidants and anti-inflammatory properties.
- **Paprika**: Adds flavor and contains antioxidants that help fight inflammation.
- **Tomatoes**: Rich in lycopene, an antioxidant that helps reduce inflammation.
- **Coconut Milk**: Provides healthy fats and antioxidants that support overall health and reduce inflammation.
- **Cilantro and Lemon**: Add flavor and provide antioxidants and anti-inflammatory properties.

This recipe includes ingredients known for their anti-inflammatory properties.

2. Quinoa and Vegetable Pilaf

Ingredients:

- 1 cup quinoa, rinsed
- 2 tablespoons olive oil
- 1 onion, finely chopped
- 2 cloves garlic, minced
- 1 bell pepper, diced
- 1 zucchini, diced
- 1 carrot, diced
- 1 teaspoon ground turmeric
- 1 teaspoon ground cumin
- 1/2 teaspoon smoked paprika
- 2 cups vegetable broth
- 1 cup frozen peas (select peas with no additives)
- Salt and pepper to taste
- Fresh parsley, chopped (for garnish)
- Lemon wedges (for serving)

Instructions:

1. In a large pot, heat the olive oil over medium heat.
2. Add the onion and garlic. Sauté until fragrant and the onion is translucent.
3. Add the bell pepper, zucchini, and carrot. Cook for another 5 minutes.
4. Stir in the quinoa, turmeric, cumin, and smoked paprika. Cook for 1 minute to toast the spices.

5. Add the vegetable broth and bring to a boil.
6. Reduce the heat, cover, and let it simmer for 15 minutes or until the quinoa is cooked and the liquid is absorbed.
7. Stir in the frozen peas and cook for another 5 minutes.
8. Season with salt and pepper to taste.
9. Serve hot, garnished with fresh parsley and lemon wedges.

Ingredient Benefits:

- **Quinoa**: High in protein, fiber, and essential amino acids, supporting digestive health and reducing inflammation.
- **Olive Oil**: Contains healthy fats and antioxidants that reduce inflammation.
- **Onion and Garlic**: Rich in antioxidants and sulfur compounds that have anti-inflammatory and immune-boosting properties.
- **Bell Pepper, Zucchini, and Carrot**: Rich in vitamins, minerals, and antioxidants that support overall health and reduce inflammation.
- **Turmeric**: Contains curcumin, a powerful anti-inflammatory compound.
- **Cumin**: Provides antioxidants and anti-inflammatory properties.
- **Smoked Paprika**: Adds flavor and contains antioxidants that help fight inflammation.
- **Vegetable Broth**: Provides flavor without the inflammatory compounds found in meat-based broths.
- **Frozen Peas**: High in fiber, vitamins, and antioxidants that support overall health and reduce inflammation.
- **Parsley and Lemon**: Add flavor and provide antioxidants and anti-inflammatory properties.

This recipe includes ingredients known for their anti-inflammatory properties.

3. Chickpea and Spinach Stew

Ingredients:

- 1 tablespoon olive oil
- 1 onion, finely chopped
- 3 cloves garlic, minced
- 1 teaspoon ground cumin
- 1 teaspoon ground coriander
- 1 teaspoon smoked paprika
- 1/2 teaspoon ground turmeric
- 1 can (14.5 oz) diced tomatoes
- 2 cans (14.5 oz each) chickpeas, drained and rinsed
- 4 cups vegetable broth
- 4 cups fresh spinach, roughly chopped
- Salt and pepper to taste
- Fresh cilantro, chopped (for garnish)
- Lemon wedges (for serving)

Instructions:

1. In a large pot, heat the olive oil over medium heat.
2. Add the onion and garlic. Sauté until fragrant and the onion is translucent.
3. Stir in the cumin, coriander, smoked paprika, and turmeric. Cook for 1 minute until the spices are fragrant.
4. Add the diced tomatoes, chickpeas, and vegetable broth. Bring to a boil.

5. Reduce the heat and let it simmer for 20 minutes to allow the flavors to meld.
6. Stir in the fresh spinach and cook until wilted, about 2–3 minutes.
7. Season with salt and pepper to taste.
8. Serve hot, garnished with fresh cilantro and lemon wedges.

Ingredient Benefits:

- **Lentils, Quinoa, and Chickpeas**: These plant-based proteins are high in fiber, vitamins, and minerals, which support overall health and reduce inflammation.
- **Turmeric**: Contains curcumin, a powerful anti-inflammatory compound.
- **Olive Oil**: Rich in monounsaturated fats and antioxidants, it has anti-inflammatory properties.
- **Vegetables (Carrots, Celery, Bell Pepper, Zucchini, Spinach)**: Packed with vitamins, minerals, and antioxidants that support overall health and reduce inflammation.
- **Garlic and Ginger**: Both have anti-inflammatory and antioxidant properties.
- **Coconut Milk**: Provides a creamy texture and healthy fats without dairy.

4. Mexican Black Beans and Rice

Ingredients:

- 1 cup brown rice
- 1 tablespoon olive oil
- 1 onion, finely chopped

- 2 cloves garlic, minced
- 1 bell pepper, diced
- 1 teaspoon ground cumin
- 1 teaspoon smoked paprika
- 1 teaspoon ground coriander
- 1/2 teaspoon chili powder
- 1 can (14.5 oz) black beans, drained and rinsed
- 1 can (14.5 oz) diced tomatoes
- 2 cups vegetable broth
- 1 cup frozen corn
- Salt and pepper to taste
- Fresh cilantro, chopped (for garnish)
- Lime wedges (for serving)

Instructions:

1. Cook the brown rice according to package instructions.
2. Heat the olive oil over medium heat in a large skillet.
3. Add the onion and garlic. Sauté until fragrant and the onion is translucent.
4. Add the bell pepper and cook for another 5 minutes.
5. Stir in the cumin, smoked paprika, ground coriander, and chili powder. Cook for 1 minute until the spices are fragrant.
6. Add the black beans, diced tomatoes, and vegetable broth. Bring to a boil.
7. Reduce the heat and let it simmer for 10–15 minutes or until the mixture thickens slightly.
8. Stir in the cooked rice and frozen corn and cook until heated through.
9. Season with salt and pepper to taste.
10. Serve hot, garnished with fresh cilantro and lime wedges.

Ingredient Benefits:

- **Brown Rice**: A whole grain rich in fiber, vitamins, and minerals, which helps reduce inflammation and support digestive health.
- **Olive Oil**: Contains monounsaturated fats and antioxidants that have anti-inflammatory properties.
- **Onion**: High in antioxidants, particularly quercetin, which has anti-inflammatory effects.
- **Garlic**: Contains sulfur compounds that have anti-inflammatory and immune-boosting properties.
- **Bell Pepper**: Rich in vitamins A and C, antioxidants that reduce inflammation and support immune function.
- **Ground Cumin**: Contains anti-inflammatory compounds and helps improve digestion.
- **Smoked Paprika**: Adds flavor and contains antioxidants that help fight inflammation.
- **Ground Coriander**: Contains antioxidants and has anti-inflammatory properties.
- **Chili Powder**: Contains capsaicin, which has anti-inflammatory and pain-relieving properties.
- **Black Beans**: High in fiber, protein, and antioxidants, beans help reduce inflammation and support overall health.
- **Diced Tomatoes**: Rich in lycopene, an antioxidant that helps reduce inflammation.
- **Vegetable Broth**: Provides flavor without the inflammatory compounds found in meat-based broths.
- **Frozen Corn**: Contains fiber, vitamins, and antioxidants that support overall health.
- **Fresh Cilantro**: Contains antioxidants and anti-inflammatory compounds.

- **Lime Wedges**: Rich in vitamin C, which has antioxidant properties.

5. Mediterranean Chickpeas and Rice

Ingredients:

- 1 cup basmati rice
- 1 tablespoon olive oil
- 1 onion, finely chopped
- 3 cloves garlic, minced
- 1 teaspoon ground cumin
- 1 teaspoon ground turmeric
- 1 teaspoon ground coriander
- 1/2 teaspoon ground cinnamon
- 1 can (14.5 oz) chickpeas, drained and rinsed
- 1 can (14.5 oz) diced tomatoes
- 2 cups vegetable broth
- 1/2 cup kalamata olives, sliced
- 1/4 cup fresh parsley, chopped
- Salt and pepper to taste
- Lemon wedges (for serving)

Instructions:

1. Cook the basmati rice according to package instructions.
2. Heat the olive oil over medium heat in a large skillet.
3. Add the onion and garlic. Sauté until fragrant and the onion is translucent.
4. Stir in the cumin, turmeric, ground coriander, and cinnamon. Cook for 1 minute until the spices are fragrant.

5. Add the chickpeas, diced tomatoes, and vegetable broth. Bring to a boil.
6. Reduce the heat and let it simmer for 10–15 minutes or until the mixture thickens slightly.
7. Stir in the cooked rice, kalamata olives, and fresh parsley. Cook until heated through.
8. Season with salt and pepper to taste.
9. Serve hot, garnished with lemon wedges.

Ingredient Benefits:

- **Basmati Rice**: A whole grain with a low glycemic index that provides steady energy and helps reduce inflammation.
- **Olive Oil**: Contains monounsaturated fats and antioxidants that have anti-inflammatory properties.
- **Onion**: High in antioxidants, particularly quercetin, which has anti-inflammatory effects.
- **Garlic**: Contains sulfur compounds that have anti-inflammatory and immune-boosting properties.
- **Ground Cumin**: Contains anti-inflammatory compounds and helps improve digestion.
- **Ground Turmeric**: Contains curcumin, a powerful anti-inflammatory compound.
- **Ground Coriander**: Contains antioxidants and has anti-inflammatory properties.
- **Ground Cinnamon**: Contains antioxidants and has anti-inflammatory properties.
- **Chickpeas**: High in fiber, protein, and antioxidants, chickpeas help reduce inflammation and support overall health.
- **Diced Tomatoes**: Rich in lycopene, an antioxidant that helps reduce inflammation.

- **Vegetable Broth**: Provides flavor without the inflammatory compounds found in meat-based broths.
- **Kalamata Olives**: Rich in healthy fats and antioxidants that support heart health and reduce inflammation.
- **Fresh Parsley**: Contains antioxidants and anti-inflammatory compounds.
- **Lemon Wedges**: Rich in vitamin C, which has antioxidant properties.

6. Caribbean Red Beans and Rice

Ingredients:

- 1 cup long-grain brown rice
- 1 tablespoon coconut oil
- 1 onion, finely chopped
- 2 cloves garlic, minced
- 1 teaspoon ground allspice
- 1 teaspoon dried thyme
- 1/2 teaspoon smoked paprika
- 1 can (14.5 oz) red kidney beans, drained and rinsed
- 1 can (14.5 oz) coconut milk
- 1 cup vegetable broth
- 1 bell pepper, diced
- 1 cup frozen peas (select peas with no additives)
- Salt and pepper to taste
- Fresh cilantro, chopped (for garnish)
- Lime wedges (for serving)

Instructions:

1. Cook the brown rice according to package instructions.
2. Heat the coconut oil over medium heat in a large skillet,
3. Add the onion and garlic. Sauté until fragrant and the onion is translucent.
4. Stir in the allspice, thyme, and smoked paprika. Cook for 1 minute until the spices are fragrant.
5. Add the kidney beans, coconut milk, and vegetable broth. Bring to a boil.
6. Reduce the heat and let it simmer for 10–15 minutes or until the mixture thickens slightly.
7. Stir in the cooked rice, bell pepper, and frozen peas. Cook until heated through.
8. Season with salt and pepper to taste.
9. Serve hot, garnished with fresh cilantro and lime wedges.

Ingredient Benefits:

- **Beans (Black Beans, Chickpeas, Kidney Beans)**: High in fiber, protein, and antioxidants, beans help reduce inflammation and support overall health.
- **Brown Rice and Basmati Rice**: Whole grains provide fiber, vitamins, and minerals, promoting digestive health and reducing inflammation.
- **Olive Oil and Coconut Oil**: Healthy fats with anti-inflammatory properties.
- **Vegetables (Onion, Garlic, Bell Pepper, Tomatoes, Corn, Peas)**: Packed with vitamins, minerals, and antioxidants that support overall health and reduce inflammation.

- **Spices (Cumin, Turmeric, Coriander, Paprika, Allspice, Thyme)**: These spices not only add flavor but also have anti-inflammatory and antioxidant properties.
- **Long-Grain Brown Rice**: A whole grain rich in fiber, vitamins, and minerals, which helps reduce inflammation and support digestive health.
- **Coconut Oil**: Contains medium-chain triglycerides (MCTs) and antioxidants that have anti-inflammatory properties.
- **Onion**: High in antioxidants, particularly quercetin, which has anti-inflammatory effects.
- **Garlic**: Contains sulfur compounds that have anti-inflammatory and immune-boosting properties.
- **Ground Allspice**: Contains antioxidants and anti-inflammatory compounds.
- **Dried Thyme**: Contains antioxidants and has anti-inflammatory properties.
- **Smoked Paprika**: Adds flavor and contains antioxidants that help fight inflammation.
- **Red Kidney Beans**: High in fiber, protein, and antioxidants, beans help reduce inflammation and support overall health.
- **Coconut Milk**: Provides healthy fats and antioxidants and has anti-inflammatory properties.
- **Vegetable Broth**: Provides flavor without the inflammatory compounds found in meat-based broths.
- **Bell Pepper**: Rich in vitamins A and C, antioxidants that reduce inflammation and support immune function.
- **Frozen Peas**: High in fiber, vitamins, and antioxidants that support overall health and reduce inflammation.
- **Fresh Cilantro**: Contains antioxidants and anti-inflammatory compounds.

- **Lime Wedges**: Rich in vitamin C, which has antioxidant properties.

These one-pot dishes are easy to prepare and offer a variety of flavors while supporting an anti-inflammatory diet.

References and Resources

1. Harvard Health Publishing. (n.d.). Understanding acute and chronic inflammation. Harvard Health. Retrieved June 13, 2024, from https://www.health.harvard.edu/staying-healthy/understanding-acute-and-chronic-inflammation
2. Harvard T.H. Chan School of Public Health. (n.d.). Diet review: Anti-inflammatory diet. The Nutrition Source. Retrieved June 13, 2024, from https://nutritionsource.hsph.harvard.edu/healthy-weight/diet-reviews/anti-inflammatory-diet/
3. MD Anderson Cancer Center. (n.d.). 3 myths about inflammation. Retrieved June 13, 2024, from https://www.mdanderson.org/cancerwise/3-myths-about-inflammation-and-cancer.h00-159301467.html
4. University of Chicago Medicine. (2020, September). What foods cause or reduce inflammation? UChicago Medicine. Retrieved June 13, 2024, from https://www.uchicagomedicine.org/en/forefront/gastrointestinal-articles/2020/september/what-foods-cause-or-reduce-inflammation
5. Mayo Clinic Health System. (n.d.). Want to ease chronic inflammation? Start with your grocery list. Retrieved June 13, 2024, from https://www.mayoclinichealthsystem.org/hometown-health/speaking-of-health/want-to-ease-chronic-inflammation
6. U.S. Food and Drug Administration. (n.d.). How to understand and use the nutrition facts label. Retrieved June 13, 2024, from https://www.fda.gov/food/nutrition-facts-label/how-understand-and-use-nutrition-facts-label
7. Zhang, R., Li, Y., Zhang, A. L., Zhou, K., & Zhao, G. (2020). The gut microbiota and inflammation: An overview. PMC. Retrieved June 13, 2024, from https://www.ncbi.nlm.nih.gov/pmc/articles/PMC7589951/
8. Meal Village. (n.d.). Mastering macros for a balanced diet: Your essential guide. Retrieved June 13, 2024, from https://www.mealvillage.com/blog/macronutrients-for-a-balanced-diet.jsp
9. EatingWell. (n.d.). 30-day anti-inflammatory diet meal plan. Retrieved June 13, 2024, from https://www.eatingwell.com/article/7866186/30-day-anti-inflammatory-meal-plan/
10. Experience Life by Life Time. (n.d.). 5 expert meal prep tips that save you time. Retrieved June 13, 2024, from https://experiencelife.lifetime.life/article/5-expert-meal-prep-tips-that-save-you-time/
11. BBC Good Food. (n.d.). 7 days of healthy budget family meals. Retrieved June

13, 2024, from https://www.bbcgoodfood.com/howto/guide/seven-nights-healthy-budget-family-suppers

12. An, J. Y., & Fiocco, A. J. (2021). The effect of an anti-inflammatory diet on chronic pain. PMC. Retrieved June 13, 2024, from https://www.ncbi.nlm.nih.gov/pmc/articles/PMC10381948/

13. Institute for Integrative Nutrition. (n.d.). Six anti-inflammatory holiday recipes. Retrieved June 13, 2024, from https://www.integrativenutrition.com/blog/antiinflammatory-holiday-recipes

14. Rethink Nourishment. (n.d.). How to host people with dietary restrictions. Retrieved June 13, 2024, from https://www.rethinknourishment.com/blog/how-to-host-people-dietary-restrictions

15. Rosen, E. (2022, January 10). How to mindfully manage your food cravings. The New York Times. Retrieved June 13, 2024, from https://www.nytimes.com/2022/01/10/well/eat/food-cravings-strategies.html

16. Scripps Health. (n.d.). Six keys to reducing inflammation. Retrieved June 13, 2024, from https://www.scripps.org/news_items/4232-six-keys-to-reducing-inflammation#:

17. Irwin, M. R., & Opp, M. (2012). Sleep loss and inflammation. PMC. Retrieved June 13, 2024, from https://www.ncbi.nlm.nih.gov/pmc/articles/PMC3548567/

18. Goodwin Living. (n.d.). Fight inflammation by staying hydrated. Retrieved June 13, 2024, from https://goodwinliving.org/blog/fight-inflammation-by-staying-hydrated/

19. Link, R. (n.d.). 10 supplements that fight inflammation. Healthline. Retrieved June 13, 2024, from https://www.healthline.com/nutrition/anti-inflammatory-supplements

20. Gottlieb, B. (n.d.). What you should know about nightshades and arthritis. Arthritis Foundation. Retrieved June 13, 2024, from https://www.arthritis.org/health-wellness/healthy-living/nutrition/anti-inflammatory/how-nightshades-affect-arthritis

21. Haldar, S. (2022). 17 science-based benefits of omega-3 fatty acids. Healthline. Retrieved June 13, 2024, from https://www.healthline.com/nutrition/17-health-benefits-of-omega-3#:

22. Zelman, K. M. (n.d.). 8 diet motivation tips for success. WebMD. Retrieved June 13, 2024, from https://www.webmd.com/obesity/features/diet-motivation-tips

23. Harvard Health Publishing. (n.d.). Foods that fight inflammation. Harvard Health. Retrieved June 13, 2024, from https://www.health.harvard.edu/staying-healthy/foods-that-fight-inflammation

24. Office of Disease Prevention and Health Promotion. (n.d.). Eat Healthy, Be Active Community Workshops. U.S. Department of Health & Human Services. Retrieved June 13, 2024, from https://health.gov/our-work/nutrition-physical-

activity/dietary-guidelines/previous-dietary-guidelines/2015/eat-healthy-be-active-community-workshops.
25. Dreher, M. L., & Davenport, A. J. (2013). Hass avocado composition and potential health effects. *Critical Reviews in Food Science and Nutrition, 53*(7), 738-750. https://doi.org/10.1080/10408398.2011.556759
26. Physicians Committee for Responsible Medicine. (n.d.). Plant-based diet for beginners. Retrieved from https://www.pcrm.org/good-nutrition/plant-based-diets
27. National Institutes of Health. (2020). Spinach. Retrieved from https://ods.od.nih.gov/factsheets/Spinach-HealthProfessional/
28. Mahdavi, R., Nikniaz, L., Rafraf, M., & Jouyban, A. (2011). Determination and comparison of the total polyphenol contents of fresh and cooked vegetables. *Food and Nutrition Sciences, 2*(2), 159-166. https://doi.org/10.4236/fns.2011.22021
29. Slimestad, R., Fossen, T., & Vågen, I. M. (2007). Onions: A source of unique dietary flavonoids. *Journal of Agricultural and Food Chemistry, 55*(25), 10067-10080. https://doi.org/10.1021/jf0712503
30. Covas, M. I., Nyyssönen, K., Poulsen, H. E., Kaikkonen, J., Zunft, H. J., Kiesewetter, H., ... & Fito, M. (2006). The effect of polyphenols in olive oil on heart disease risk factors: A randomized trial. *Annals of Internal Medicine, 145*(5), 333-341. https://doi.org/10.7326/0003-4819-145-5-200609050-00006
31. Pedreschi, F., & Mariotti-Celis, M. S. (2015). Avocado oil: Production and market demand. *Trends in Food Science & Technology, 44*(2), 172-181. https://doi.org/10.1016/j.tifs.2015.04.006

www.ingramcontent.com/pod-product-compliance
Lightning Source LLC
LaVergne TN
LVHW041809060526
838201LV00046B/1181